THE HEALTH SERVICES OF IRELAND

BRENDAN HENSEY

COMPLETELY REVISED 4th EDITION

INSTITUTE OF PUBLIC ADMINISTRATION

ISBN 0 906980 87 9   Hardback

ISBN 0 906980 92 5   Paperback

Published by the
Institute of Public Administration
57–61 Lansdowne Road
Dublin 4
Ireland

First Published 1959
Second Edition 1972
Third Edition 1979
Fourth Edition 1988
Reprinted 1990

Origination in 11/12 point Baskerville by Dublin University Press Limited
Printed by the Leinster Leader Limited, Naas

Contents

Do Máire, mo bean céile

Foreword

As was the case with earlier editions of *The Health Services of Ireland*, the primary purpose of this book is to describe the health services and the system within which they are organised. As a prelude to this description, an account is given of the origins of the services. To understand the present calls for some knowledge of the past.

In the preparation of this edition, there has been considerable re-writing of the last edition and much new material has been included. I am indebted to the Department of Health for supplying much of the basis for this material. The secretary, Liam Flanagan, generously agreed to the department's co-operation in my establishing the facts. I had discussions with several of my former colleagues in the department. All were most helpful. My thanks are especially due to Denis Cronin, who co-ordinated my contacts and himself supplied answers to several of my queries. Donal Devitt, Tony Enright, Paul Kelly, Michael Lyons, John Quinn and Tadgh Tansley were all most helpful in their own fields. A debt is due too to two other members of the department, Ruth Barrington and Joe Robins, whose books give much fuller treatments than I do of the parts of the services which they cover, not only for the use of their books as references but also for helpful comments on the points which I raised with them. I also received valuable assistance from Philip Berman (European Association of Programmes in Health Services Studies), Vincent Breheny (An Bord Altranais), Joe Cahill (Pharmaceutical Society of Ireland), Dr Emer Shelley (Kilkenny Health Project) and Michael Stanley (Bord na Radharcmhastoiri) and I would also like to thank Dr Tom Murphy for his advice on part of the text.

Once again, I wish to acknowledge the contribution of Jim O'Donnell and his staff in the Institute of Public

Administration. The editing and the processing of my manuscript was guided by the skilled hands of Iain MacAulay. I thank him and the others involved.

In the introduction to the first edition of *The Health Services of Ireland,* in 1959, I wrote:

> I have limited the scope of this book so as to relate it only to the services organised by public authorities, but it has been no part of my design either to defend or criticise these services as such, or their operation. While the work is, therefore, intended only to describe, it is well to make it clear that, if any opinion can be inferred from it, it does not necessarily represent official policy. As a defending counsel might put it, I express no opinion and any opinion I do express is all my own.

This cagey saver was made by a writer who was then a middle-grade officer in the Department of Health, with hopes of rising higher. Now, at more than six years' remove from the department, no such saver seems called for. While the present edition remains essentially descriptive, description is laced with comment. It is hardly necessary for me to state that, at this remove, any comment represents my personal views, without any seal of official approval.

Brendan Hensey
March 1988

CHAPTER ONE

The growth of the health services
– the nineteenth century

'Health services' may be defined as those services under which public authorities arrange for the diagnosis, prevention and treatment of human illness. The purpose of this book is to explain what the health services are, how they originated, how they are operated, who is entitled to them and how much they cost. It is concerned with the relationships of the state and public bodies with, on the one hand, the medical profession and other health professions and, on the other hand, the general public. These relationships have developed from the increasing recognition of the fact that simple private arrangements between individual practitioners and patients could not offer to the general public the full benefits of an expanding medical science. Some form of organisation of health services became essential once discoveries in that science began to move out of the fields of homely palliatives and simple empirical cures.

A number of the institutions from which our present health services were derived had their roots in the eighteenth century. The system of public voluntary hospitals originated in the early decades of that century and the first hospital for the insane, St Patrick's Hospital, was opened in Dublin in 1757. These institutions were founded primarily by private charity but, in varying degrees, were aided from public funds. The second half of the eighteenth century saw the humble and impoverished commencement of the local authority

1

hospital system with the establishment of county infirmaries and fever hospitals under the management of committees on which the public authorities were represented.

However, overall the eighteenth century bequeathed to the nineteenth little by way of resources for health services. The latter part of the eighteenth century was not conducive to thought and action for the betterment of such services, being a period of bitter conflict and unrest, culminating in the insurrection of 1798, its harsh suppression and the passing of the Act of Union with Britain. After the year 1800, responsibility for lawmaking and administration was concentrated in London. Basic decisions in the development of services in Ireland were made there. So, the general influences moulding the outlooks of successive United Kingdom governments in the nineteenth century formed the basis of decisions on the development of health services in Ireland. The early part of the century carried over the laissez-faire economic and social theories of the eighteenth century but, as the new century wore on, these theories became diluted by the assimilation of new social theories which recognised an increasing role for the state in social development.

THE NINETEENTH CENTURY SERVICES

Hospitals, infirmaries and workhouses
During the nineteenth century, the voluntary hospital system continued to grow. Several new hospitals, based on lay philanthropy, were added, mainly in Dublin, and there were new foundations of major hospitals by religious orders in Dublin and Cork. These voluntary hospitals are itemised in chapter eleven.

Outside the areas served by the voluntary hospitals, there was no comparable general hospital system. By the eighteen-thirties, about twenty county infirmaries had been opened, as well as about seventy fever hospitals, but these were on the whole quite inadequate and were poorly financed. The origins of our general hospital system outside the cities lay

2

rather in the new institutions set up under the Poor Relief (Ireland) Act, 1838.

That act put a duty on the Poor Law Commissioners to accommodate the destitute in workhouses. About one hundred of these were built and opened within the four years following the passage of the act[1]. The primary duty of the poor law guardians described on page 10 was in the maintenance of the poor and not in their medical care but, as many of the inmates could be expected to need such care from time to time, the design of the workhouse buildings allowed for the incorporation of infirmaries.

The workhouses were planned to be grim and strictly functional, deliberately so, as it was a tenet of the poor law to discourage all but the absolutely destitute from partaking of its benefits. The public authorities of the day had no vision of these institutions becoming hospitals but, during the nineteenth century, hospital services were increasingly based on workhouses and many of the workhouse buildings were to become part of the basis of the county hospital system in the twentieth century.

The dispensary service

In the eighteenth century, services were provided in some areas by general practitioners at dispensaries and, because of the inadequacy of the county infirmaries, the grand juries were given authority early in the nineteenth century to contribute towards the cost of such services. In the following years, many districts were provided with dispensaries, but the service did not become universal until the second half of the century.

This was effected by the Poor Relief (Ireland) Act, 1851, which placed a duty on the Irish Poor Law Commissioners to see that the boards of guardians provided dispensaries and appointed medical officers. Each poor law union was divided into a number of dispensary districts. The dispensary doctor was given the duty of attending, without charge, to the sick poor in his district, these being identified through the issue of 'red tickets' by authorised persons in the poor law system.

He was entitled to attend to those outside this class as a private practitioner. Usually the dispensary doctor himself issued any medicines he thought necessary for his public patients, requisitioning supplies from the public authorities, but apothecaries were employed in a small number of districts. The development of the dispensary system helped to make up for the deficiencies in the infirmaries and did ensure a spread of medical care in rural Ireland. However, the quality of this care was not always good. Dr Robert Collis in *The State of Medicine in Ireland* [2] described the service as it was in the late nineteenth century:

> It was not until 1806 that a medical service for the poor was introduced – The Irish Dispensary System. At first it was very incomplete, but was steadily expanded till, in 1887, there were 721 dispensary districts, having 1,093 stations, 808 medical officers, 40 apothecaries and 268 midwives. The average salary at that time was £118 a year. Each dispensary was governed by a board of guardians. A Carmichael Essayist of the time describes these committees of guardians as among 'the lower forms of life'. The guardians in those days elected the doctor; every form of graft, religious fanaticism and nepotism was the rule in these elections. The problems of the dispensary doctor of those days were truly appalling. He had to trudge long miles on foot, and ride through bogs and up watercourses to reach his patients. His pay was hopelessly inadequate and he had no regular pension so that he hung on long after he was fit for work. Many died of overwork and quite a few of drink. It was a hopeless and thankless job, and the bad name 'dispensary doctor' – 'Oh, he's just a dispensary doctor' – came from those days, for naturally the patients suffered more than anybody else. The whole system was built up on the necessity to bring some medical treatment to those who were too poor to pay for it and, like the workhouse system, its whole basis was pauperism.

4

Registration of births, deaths and marriages

The development of the dispensary system facilitated the introduction of the civil registration of births and deaths and the extension of the system for the registration of marriages. In 1863, the dispensary doctors were made registrars of births and deaths and of Catholic marriages (other marriages were registered under a different earlier system). The dispensary doctor, in his capacity of registrar, was subject to a superintendent registrar, who was usually the clerk of the poor law union. The entire system was made subject to the Registrar-General, an autonomous official appointed by the Lord Lieutenant[3]. This important outcrop of the poor law services was to be the source in later years of many of the vital statistics which formed the basis of plans for further development in the health services and other services.

Lunacy and idiocy

Dr Joseph Robins in *Fools and Mad*[4] graphically describes the condition at the commencement of the nineteenth century of the unfortunate sector of the people who were designated as lunatics and idiots. Theories and policies on their care and confinement were harsh. Those not left to wander the roads were confined—often in chains—in gaols or houses of industry (institutions set up in the eighteenth century to incarcerate beggars). It was generally accepted in that century that insanity was caused by moral weakness and called for harsh treatment for its control and cure. Hence, few saw anything wrong with the punitive treatment given in the institutions of the day.

The early nineteenth century witnessed increasing acceptance of a new outlook on mental abnormality which viewed it as a disease which was sometimes curable and which should always be seen as a condition warranting sympathetic care. It became official policy for the insane to be taken out of the gaols and houses of industry and accommodated in lunatic asylums. Legislation was passed for the establishment of these. The first, the Richmond Asylum in Dublin (now St Brendan's Hospital) was opened in 1815 and in the following sixty years district lunatic asylums were established over the whole country. A number of private asylums were also built.

As well as catering for the mentally ill, the district asylums had, from the beginning, admitted those whom we would now define as mentally handicapped and who were at the time generally described as idiots, or *daoine le Dia*. Because of their incurable condition, few of these could be discharged and, to use an inelegant modern term, the asylums tended to become 'silted-up' with them. Accordingly, when the workhouses were built after 1838, accommodation was specially provided in them for a class described as 'idiots etc'. This questionable decision had the result that, by the end of the century, most of the institutionalised mentally handicapped were being kept in the workhouses. At that time only about one-tenth of those in the district lunatic asylums were classified as idiots.

Robins summarises the position at the end of the century thus:

The position of lunacy in Ireland at the beginning of the twentieth century can be summarised briefly. There were about 21,000 insane persons of all categories in care, either in asylums or workhouses, and the number was continuing to rise. Thousands of others, mainly idiots, resided in their own homes or led a largely vagrant life. Those in the institutions were receiving care rather than treatment. Isolation and safe custody had taken over from moral treatment. Because its clinical dimension appeared to be minimal the management of lunacy was now seen as only peripherally involved with medicine and it operated without any real links with the care of the physically ill. This segregation of mental illness itself helped to strengthen the stigma associated in many minds with the asylum patient. There was, consequently, a ready public acquiescence in the policy of confining the problem of insanity behind high walls both in the literal and the figurative sense and no great inclination on the part of anyone to spend more money on improving the quality of care. There were, however, important scientific, political and administrative developments taking place which, in differing ways, would influence the care of the insane in Ireland[5].

Not a very enthusiastic endorsement of progress made, but was not the picture much better than it had been at the end of the eighteenth century?

Preventive services

The frequent occurrence of the pestilences which were common in Ireland in the nineteenth century spurred the authorities to spasmodic efforts to control them and alleviate their effects. Temporary commissioners of health were, for example, appointed at the time of the Great Famine and these acted in some respects through the local boards of guardians. Anything done at this time was unsystematic and, with the exception of smallpox vaccination, which was introduced in 1858, none of the measures of that time could be regarded as a forerunner of our present preventive services. It was not until the work of Chadwick, Simon and others in Britain punched home the connection between environment and infectious diseases and led to the introduction there of a systemised effective sanitary law, that serious attention was given to the development of the sanitary services and the preventive health services in Ireland.

Sanitary services could not realistically be organised except by public authorities; neither could the preventive services which were ancillary to them. Thus, at a time when curative medicine, inside and outside hospitals, was still largely left to individuals and private organisations, the preventive services became a clear-cut responsibility of the public authorities. The earlier piecemeal efforts were drawn together and codified in the Public Health (Ireland) Act, 1878. This was closely modelled on an earlier English act and was designed mainly to provide a single body of law on the provision of water supplies, sewerage works and similar

services. However, a small part of this code related to health
services as we have defined them, and this was until 1947
the legal basis for a considerable sector of the health services.

The most important provisions in the act from the point
of view of the health services were those under which power
was given to the Local Government Board to make regulations
to prevent the spread of infectious diseases. Food hygiene
controls also originated in this act, which contained
prohibitions on the sale of food which was 'diseased,
contaminated, or otherwise unfit for human consumption.'
The dispensary doctors became holders under this act of an
additional office of medical officer of health, with duties
related mainly to the control of infectious diseases. In the
cities of Dublin, Cork, Limerick and Waterford, medical
superintendent officers of health were appointed to supervise
and co-ordinate the work of the local medical officers of
health, but in the rural areas the co-ordination and supervision
of the work of the district medical officers of health remained
entirely with the medical inspectors of the Local Government
Board.

ADMINISTRATION

Central administration
In the early nineteenth century there was no central authority
established specifically for the administration of health
services. Such functions as fell to be discharged at the centre
in relation to the lunatic asylums and the other services
which existed then were discharged by the Lord Lieutenant
or his subordinates. The year 1838 saw the first departure
from this. The Poor Relief (Ireland) Act of that year
established a tightly organised administration for the relief of
the poor, which became responsible for the development of a
number of services. Substantial powers were reserved under
this legislation to the central authority, which in the first
instance was the English Poor Law Commissioners. While
this body accomplished its initial task of equipping the

country with workhouses, the remoteness of the commissioners from the work in Ireland made the arrangement an unsatisfactory one for the continued operation of the services. In 1847, the Irish Poor Law Commissioners were appointed to take over the functions of the English commissioners[6].

The Irish Poor Law Commissioners were appointed by the Queen. Their task was to ensure uniformity in the poor law services and they exercised very detailed control over the local authorities providing them. Their field of action was, however, limited to the poor law services. Other local government services (and in particular the sanitary services) were developing at this time and the need grew for a central co-ordinating authority. The Royal Sanitary Commission of 1869 reported in favour of a government-appointed board to take over the functions of the Irish Poor Law Commissioners and be responsible also for supervising the other services. The Irish Local Government Board was, in accordance with this recommendation, established in 1872[7] and remained the administrative authority for the local government and health services until the third decade of the twentieth century.

The Irish Local Government Board consisted of five members, under the presidency of the Chief Secretary to the Lord Lieutenant. One of the members was required to be medically qualified. With one exception, the services described above came within the board's jurisdiction. The exception was the care of the insane, which remained directly under the Lord Lieutenant. Under him, inspectors of lunacy had considerable autonomy in the supervision of this service.

Local administration
Health service administration evolved within the local government system, for which the nineteenth century was a period of considerable change and development. The trend in local government was towards greater uniformity in the pattern of authorities and a widening of the franchise on which they were elected. Each of the classes of authorities then established and developed was responsible for a number of local services but, in the allocation of these, the health

services were not viewed as a unit. There was no apparent endeavour to rationalise and co-ordinate at a local level the administration of the health services then developing. Generally speaking, each service, as it was introduced, was made the responsibility of whichever of the existing sets of local authorities was considered to be the most convenient. In stating this, a reservation should be made for the mental treatment service. The maintenance and financing of lunatic asylums remained the responsibility of committees of management specially appointed for the purpose by the central authority. These committees were not truly local authorities in the present day meaning of the term, but they were at the time the only group of bodies specially created for the provision of a health service.

During this period two main sets of local authorities became concerned with the provision of the services – the boards of guardians and the sanitary authorities. The boards of guardians were the local agents of the Poor Law Commissioners, having come into being under the act of 1838 referred to earlier. They were bodies with membership made up of justices of the peace and persons elected by the ratepayers. Each of these authorities served a district known as the poor law union, there being one hundred and twenty-six of these in the present area of the State.

The poor law administration had been primarily set up to provide physical necessities for paupers. Its role in the health services was at first not significant but, as indicated earlier, this role grew in importance in the decades up to 1900.

In the meantime, the sanitary authorities were evolving. These were to play an important part in developing the preventive side of the health services. There were sanitary authorities in towns since the early nineteenth century, their work consisting mainly of the provision of sewers, water-supplies, wash-houses, street lighting and other amenities conducive to health and comfort. Personal health services were at first no significant part of their functions and it was not until the sanitary administration was re-organised under the Public Health (Ireland) Acts of 1874 and 1878 that this side of their work assumed prominence. Under those acts, the existing municipal corporations and town commissioners were appointed as sanitary authorities for the larger urban areas. No special rural sanitary authorities were constituted then; the boards of guardians became the sanitary authorities for the rural areas and smaller towns.

The final change in the nineteenth century administration came with the Local Government (Ireland) Act, 1898. Under that act there were established elective county councils, urban district councils and rural district councils. The last-mentioned councils were appointed for the rural sanitary districts and took over the sanitary functions of the boards of guardians. The latter remained, however, to discharge their original functions of providing relief (including medical relief) for the poor. The county councils took over the administration (either direct or through joint committees) of the district lunatic asylums but were not otherwise concerned at the time with the health services.

Finance

The primary source of money for the health services at this time was local taxation. Some state aid was provided towards the end of the century from the estate duty grant and the licence duty grant. The estate duty grant was introduced in 1888[8]. The total grant each year was calculated as being a sum equivalent to one and one-half per cent of the net value of the property in respect of which estate duty was leviable each year. The grant was paid for a number of local services, including those of the poor law authorities. The licence duty grant, which was introduced in 1898[9], was designed to recoup specified proportions of the cost of particular items in the services. The grant was intended to meet the following:

(a) one-half of the salaries of the medical officers of workhouses and dispensaries;

(b) one-half of the salary of one trained nurse in each

11

workhouse, who was actually employed and possessed
the prescribed qualifications;

(c) the whole of the salaries of schoolmasters and
schoolmistresses in the workhouses;

(d) one-half of the cost of medicines and medical and
surgical appliances;

(e) one-half of the salaries of officers of sanitary authorities;

(f) a capitation grant for inmates of lunatic asylums at a
rate not exceeding four shillings a week.

The relative importance attached to financial incentives for
the development in the workhouses of medical and nursing
services on the one hand and schooling on the other hand
will be noticed. The funds for this grant were derived from
fees for certain local licences. If the total of these fees was
insufficient to meet the commitments, the grant for each
purpose was abated proportionately – a procedure which
called for no mean volume of calculations.

These grants had what was an advantage to the Treasury
and a disadvantage to the health administration in that they
were related to the yields of specified taxes. They could not
be used as an incentive to the local authorities for the general
development of the services as the amount available was not
sufficient to meet more than a small proportion of the total
cost of the system.

THE HEALTH PROFESSIONS

In parallel with these developments in the services and
structures for them, the health professions and their governance
had progressed. The Royal College of Physicians of Ireland
had been chartered in 1654 and the Royal College of
Surgeons received its charter in 1784 (ending the long regime
of the Guild of Barber-surgeons). These colleges and the
medical school in Trinity College had by the nineteenth
century achieved a high status internationally in the training
of medical practitioners.

Under an act passed by the Irish Parliament in 1791, the Apothecaries Hall in Dublin was given a monopolistic control on those who wished to 'open shop or practise the art and mystery of an apothecary within the Kingdom of Ireland'. The apothecary combined the roles of pharmacist and doctor (but in the latter case at a lower level than the graduates of the medical schools).

The medical register (the list of those qualified as medical practitioners) was set up under the Medical Act, 1858, which applied to the United Kingdom as a whole. The royal colleges of physicians and surgeons, the medical school of Trinity College and the Apothecaries Hall were recognised for the issue of qualifying diplomas for registration.

The apothecaries had not extended a service to cover the entire country. Hence, in 1875, their monopoly was broken to allow graduates of a newly–established Pharmaceutical Society of Ireland to 'open shop for the retail dispensing and compounding of poisons and medical prescriptions'[10]. In the case of other health professions formal structures for training and registration were to await the twentieth century. Training schools for nurses and midwives had, however, been set up in the latter part of the nineteenth century in some of the voluntary hospitals. In the lunatic asylums, however, no move had been made to upgrade the attendants who looked after the inmates.

ASSESSMENT OF THE NINETEENTH CENTURY

The legislation of the United Kingdom in the early nineteenth century was primarily geared to the needs of Britain. What was enacted for Ireland usually followed the British pattern and was not always suited to Irish conditions (the poor law is an example). The services and structures described in this chapter were designed and operated by a confident, but not always sensitive, ascendancy. However, three measures – Catholic Emancipation, the progressive widening of the electoral franchise from the eighteen-thirties and the introduction of elective local government – were to lead ultimately to more democratic control of the health services, but this did not become very evident in the nineteenth century.

The Great Famine of 1847 had led to over a million deaths and had triggered a stream of emigration which continued throughout the century (by the year 1900, the population had dropped to about half that of 1841). Those who remained on the land saw better conditions of tenure as their priority and concentrated on this. Furthermore, on a more general political level, the majority of the electorate were becoming increasingly disaffected of the Union and political activity was concentrated on the Home Rule question. These were the big issues of the second half of the century and little scope was left for political thought on social matters such as health care.

There was, however, much administrative and professional activity in the building and staffing of the workhouses and lunatic asylums, the establishment of the dispensary system, the continuing development of voluntary hospitals and the constitution of the sanitary authorities. There is no convincing evidence to show that all this activity had much effect on the health of the people by the end of the century.

The death rate in 1900, at 17.7 per 1,000 population, was little different from what it was in the eighteen-sixties and the infant mortality rate had actually increased from 95.7 per 1,000 live births in the eighteen-sixties to 99.4 per 1,000 live births in the eighteen-nineties. One achievement, however, stands out – the use of the vaccination technique discovered by Jenner in 1798 to virtually eliminate smallpox as a threat. Perhaps we should not use twentieth century standards to judge the nineteenth century. In that century the training and organisation of the medical and other health professions had been improved but knowledge, techniques and equipment were still rudimentary. For surgery, the anaesthetics which came into use were crude, blood transfusions were not available and X-ray equipment was not yet developed. Antiseptic drill in surgery was not good. The general practitioner outside the cities had little back-up from the hospitals. The medicines available to him were in no way as effective as the range available now. Dentistry meant little but painful extractions. Psychiatry had not yet emerged as a speciality.

So, how should one assess the nineteenth century developments? Some were obviously good, such as the extension of the voluntary hospital system, the creation of the sanitary authorities and, with reservations on its compulsory aspect, the smallpox vaccination scheme. Some others one might accept, with reservations, as being positive (the dispensary service and the lunatic asylums). Perhaps one should judge all these as constituting a prelude to hope for the twentieth century. One undertaking had little to commend it – the establishment of the workhouse system. The workhouses became the stark and highly visible symbols of a bad social theory uncompassionately applied. The drawings[11] below give an idea of what the exterior and part of the interior of a workhouse was like.

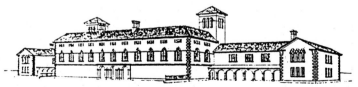

Carlow Workhouse

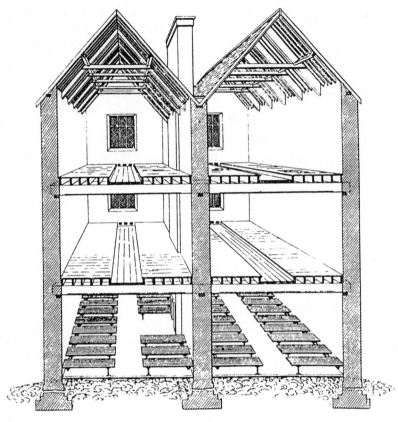

Sleeping quarters of a typical workhouse

It is perhaps a pity that one of the workhouses was not retained in its entirety and restored to its original condition (complete with straw bedding) to let the present and future generations see what life for the poor was really like in the nineteenth century, so that they might savour better the facilities of the twentieth.

NOTES ON CHAPTER ONE

1. An account of the building of the workhouses is given in an article by P.J. Meghan in *Administration*, Vol. 3, No. 1, Spring, 1955.
2. W.R.F. Collis, *The State of Medicine in Ireland* (Carmichael Prize Essay), Parkside Press, Dublin, 1943. Page 1.
3. In the present century, it became traditional for the office of Registrar-General to be held by the Secretary of the Department of Local Government and Public Health (later Health).
4. J. Robins, *Fools and Mad*, Institute of Public Administration, Dublin, 1986. Page 23 et seq.
5. Robins, op cit., page 171.
6. Under the Poor Relief (Ireland) Act, 1847.
7. Under the Irish Local Government Board Act, 1872.
8. The grant, which was originally called the probate duty grant, was first established under the Probate Duties (Ireland) Act, 1888. The name was changed to the estate duty grant by the Finance Act, 1894.
9. By section 58 of the Local Government (Ireland) Act, 1898.
10. Under the Pharmacy Act (Ireland) 1875.
11. Taken from the article by P.J. Meghan referred to above.

CHAPTER TWO

1900–1945

The main political issues were the same in the early twentieth century as in the second half of the nineteenth. The land question was to be largely answered by legislation for compulsory purchase from the landlords and the vesting of farms in the occupants. The issue of a separate parliament and administration for Ireland was unresolved. Home rule for Ireland had been conceded in legislation, but not implemented, at the outbreak of war in August 1914. After the 1916 rising and the supersession of the Irish Party by Sinn Fein, the issue became the emergence of an independent state, which was achieved by the early nineteen-twenties (with the six north-eastern counties excluded). The early part of the century was no period for concentration on social development and changes made in the health services were relatively narrow in scope.

A serious possibility for basic change did arise, however, on the National Insurance Bill in 1911. That bill was designed to establish a system of cash benefits, based on insurance, for workers when absent through illness and to combine with that a scheme of medical care primarily based on panels of general practitioners. There were divided views on the application of the bill to Ireland. The Catholic Hierarchy opposed it as being unsuited to Irish conditions. So did strong elements in the medical profession, (but the profession as a whole became ambivalent in its attitude during the passage of the bill). The Irish party's influence in the Westminster parliament was the deciding factor. The party opposed the inclusion of medical benefit in the scheme as applied to Ireland and parliament decided accordingly. The story of this non-event is recounted in full in Dr Ruth Barrington's *Health, Medicine and Politics in Ireland 1900-1970.*[1] Had the panel scheme been applied at the time in Ireland, this would have had a profound effect on the dispensary system and, perhaps, on the general development of the health care system in Ireland.

The remaining two decades of the United Kingdom regime saw no fundamental changes in the services. Some important legislation was, however, enacted. The Tuberculosis Prevention (Ireland) Act, 1908 gave the county councils and county borough corporations power to provide sanatoria and clinics and to operate services to combat tuberculosis. The same authorities were given power in 1917 to operate schemes for the prevention and treatment of venereal disease. [2] Under the Notification of Births (Extension) Act, 1915, sanitary authorities (the urban and rural district councils) were given power to make arrangements for attending to the health of expectant and nursing mothers and children under five years of age and, by the Public Health (Medical Treatment of Children) (Ireland) Act, 1919, the county councils and county borough corporations were required to provide for the medical inspection and treatment of children attending national schools. These acts marked a significant extension in the perceived role of the local authorities, particularly the county councils. Not much, however, was initiated under them before the change of regime in the nineteen-twenties.

SERVICES

Hospitals and homes
In 1920, Dail Eireann (the new Irish parliament which had been established in 1919) set about abolishing the workhouse system and gave the Minister for Local Government, Mr

William T. Cosgrave, authority to proceed with this. Dr
Barrington describes his initiative:

> The Minister dispatched envoys around the country to
> spread the new gospel of amalgamation. The young Dr
> James Ryan, later Minister for Health, was one of these.
> The level of enthusiasm varied from county to county
> and initial progress was slow. By mid-1921, however,
> many local authorities were forced to take action owing
> to the Local Government Board's withholding of grants.
> In County Galway, to take an extreme example, ten
> workhouses and the county infirmary were closed in 1921,
> while the Galway city workhouse was adapted to
> accommodate a new county hospital. David Fitzpatrick
> has described how the County Clare scheme was adopted.
> Although the county council approved amalgamation in
> principle in October 1920, it was not until June 1921
> that a scheme was drafted by a Sinn Fein organiser, Fr
> Patrick Gaynor. Two of the seven workhouses were to
> close, another converted to a sanatorium and parts of the
> remaining four reconstituted as district hospitals. The
> aged and infirm, chronic sufferers, sane epileptics and
> harmless lunatics were to be concentrated in a county
> home in Ennis. These proposals gave rise to much
> controversy. In addition to the closure and reclassification,
> the county council proposed to dismiss, without compen-
> sation, superfluous employees, to the intense annoyance
> of the council's solicitor and district clerks. The chairman
> of a board of guardians, which was to be abolished and
> lose its workhouse and officials, resigned from the county
> council in protest, warning that loyalty to the Dail had
> its limits. By mid-October 1921, the amalgamation scheme
> was provisionally accepted.
> Clare illustrates the general policy of the Department
> which in pressing for schemes of amalgamation formed
> an alliance with the county councils, stressing their role
> in supervising the entire local administration of the
> country. The Department complained that when

confronted with schemes for amalgamation of workhouses:

> Boards of Guardians not infrequently show themselves susceptible to purely parochial influences and interests which prevent them giving whole-hearted cooperation to schemes of reform and economy which are undoubtedly conceived in the best interests of the County as a whole.

> Kevin O'Higgins later explained that the main reason for local opposition to the closure of workhouses was the removal of what was considered as a local industry, the only one in some places.[3]

By this time most of the local authorities had transferred their allegiance from the Local Government Board to the Dail and they proceeded to produce the 'county schemes' as sought by the Minister. Progress was uneven but eventually a pattern for each county was agreed and their uncertain legal basis was clarified by the Local Government (Temporary Provisions) Act, 1923.

The county and district hospitals and the county homes were administered by the new boards of health and public assistance described on page 25 but the services were still governed by the Poor Relief Acts. Other priorities within the national and local finances in the nineteen-twenties precluded any major capital improvements to fit the buildings for their new roles but in the nineteen-thirties, several new county and district hospitals were built, financed mainly from the Hospitals Trust moneys referred to below. Progressive improvements were made in the quality of the staffs of local authority hospitals, but increasing specialisation in medicine and surgery led to a growth in the practice of local authorities sending some patients to the voluntary hospitals in Dublin and elsewhere. On the other hand, patients not entitled to poor relief (or public assistance, as it became known under the Public Assistance Act, 1939 which consolidated the Poor Relief Acts), began increasingly to use the local authority hospitals as paying patients.

During the nineteen-twenties, a crisis was developing in

21

the voluntary hospitals. Income was falling and, because of increased sophistication in medical and surgical equipment and techniques, costs were rising. Towards the end of the decade, some would undoubtedly have had to close their doors if the Hospitals Sweepstakes had not been authorised. These sweepstakes were based on horse-racing and commenced in 1930. They were very successful and provided funds to maintain the voluntary hospital system, as well as to build the new local authority hospitals.

The Public Hospitals Act, 1933 set up two bodies: the Hospitals Trust Board to administer the sweepstakes moneys and the Hospitals Commission to advise on the distribution of these moneys. The commission, in its first report, reviewed the hospital needs of the country generally and made recommendations for the amalgamation of some of the voluntary hospitals and for the reduction in the number of local authority hospitals. These recommendations were not well received at the time. Had they been, the problems of the nineteen-eighties might be less than they are.

The mentally ill and the mentally handicapped

These years saw no fundamental change in the system for the care of the mentally ill. In the nineteen-twenties, nomenclature changed. Lunatic asylums became mental hospitals, lunatics became patients, and attendants were replaced by nurses. As nurses became registrable by the General Nursing Council of Ireland after 1919 and better training schemes were subsequently required, there was a gradual improvement in the quality of care. However, neither the buildings nor the facilities in them were greatly changed. Very little of the sweepstakes money was allocated to mental hospitals for capital development during this period.

The mentally handicapped who were in the workhouses when the system was wound up in the nineteen-twenties were accommodated in the county homes, which made little difference to their condition at the time. The mental hospitals retained their share of the mentally handicapped. One new institution for the mentally handicapped opened—St Vincent's Home, Cabra, Dublin

Up to 1945, the nineteenth-century definitions, laws and procedures still governed the services for the care of the mentally ill. Patients were 'committed' to mental hospitals on warrants signed by peace commissioners and there was provision for nothing between detention on such warrants and complete freedom, except for a system of 'trial discharge' which did not operate well in practice. Under the Mental Treatment Act, 1945, a more flexible procedure was introduced. It provided for patients being admitted on 'reception orders' signed by medical practitioners and for procedures for temporary and voluntary admissions to mental hospitals. The use of these procedures was to improve the working of the service and make it more acceptable.

The dispensary medical service
Little change was made in the dispensary medical service during this period. The service became a responsibility of the boards of health and public assistance in 1925. Eligibility was still determined by the issue of a 'red ticket', at the time the services of the doctor were needed, by a home assistance officer or warden appointed by the local authority. Maternity care was given under this service by the dispensary doctor and a midwife was employed for each dispensary district. While the quality of the practitioners entering the service improved after their selection became the the responsibility of the Local Appointments Commission, the facilities for practice remained poor. Little was done to maintain and repair the dispensaries, which were by now old buildings, nor to furnish and equip them properly.

The preventive services
The efficiency of the preventive services was considerably improved by the appointment of the county medical officers of health under the Local Government Act, 1925, which is referred to below. The tuberculosis service and the school medical service and, in some areas, maternity and child

welfare schemes, were developed in the nineteen-twenties and thirties at a steady if unspectacular rate and this period also saw the introduction of diphtheria immunisation schemes.

The 'additional benefits' scheme
This scheme was introduced in 1942 by the National Health Insurance Society, the body then responsible for the insurance scheme under which weekly cash benefits were paid to workers disabled through ill-health. Funds surplus to the society's primary needs were made available to meet the whole or part of the cost to its members of hospital and specialist treatment (including appliances) and dental and optical treatment and appliances. The 'additional benefits' scheme operated separately from the local authority health services. Expenditure under it was limited to whatever remained after the claims for other benefits paid by the National Health Insurance Society had been met. It thus functioned intermittently and when the amount allocated to any of the additional benefits for any year was spent, the operation of that benefit ceased until the next year.

ADMINISTRATION

Central administration
No change was made by the United Kingdom government in central administration and the changes which did come in this period were incidental to the achievement of self-government. During the struggle for independence, the British authorities had maintained the Local Government Board in Dublin as the central authority, but a department of local government set up by Dail Eireann was increasingly recognised by the local authorities. For a while, therefore, there were two central authorities but, with the political settlement of the early twenties, the Local Government Board ceased to exist. Under the Ministers and Secretaries Act, 1924, the Minister for Local Government and Public Health became responsible for the services and his department took

over the role of the Local Government Board. The custom house in Dublin, which as the headquarters of the board, was burned with most of its records during the war of independence, was rebuilt and again became the centre of local government and health administration.

There were two important differences between the new central authority and the board it replaced. Firstly, it was in the charge of a minister who was no mere administrator of policy but a member of the Dail specially designated as the prime mover in the making of policy and the preparation and introduction of new health legislation. Secondly, it was responsible for all the health services, as the Minister for Local Government and Public Health had taken over the Lord Lieutenant's role in relation to the lunatic asylums.

Local administration
No significant alterations were made in local administration before 1920, the most noteworthy development of the period being that the county councils were given functions in relation to the tuberculosis and school medical services. These councils were undoubtedly the most suitable of the existing sets of authorities for those services, but their introduction to the field of general health services added one more set of authorities to the boards of guardians and sanitary authorities which already had responsibilities in that field. The achievement of self-government brought with it a number of far-reaching changes in the local administration of the services. The boards of guardians, symbolic as they were of the less beneficent side of the former administration, were abolished and were replaced in 1923 by county boards of assistance. The rural district councils were abolished in 1925[4] and except in a few areas, their sanitary functions were taken over by the boards of assistance. These bodies then became boards of health and public assistance. They were appointed by the county councils and the membership of each was made up of ten members of the parent council. The new bodies were responsible for the poor law services for the entire county, but were in charge of the sanitary and

preventive health services only for the rural districts. The urban district councils and their functions as sanitary authorities were not affected by the change. Neither were the county councils themselves. They retained responsibility for the mental health service (through joint mental hospital boards in some areas), the tuberculosis service and the school medical service.

Nothing much by way of simplification was effected by these changes, the main practical achievement being the elimination of the smaller rural local authorities (the boards of guardians and the rural district councils). However, the Local Government Act, 1925, which consolidated the new local administration, also provided for the appointment of county medical officers of health. This office was analogous to that of the medical superintendent officers of health who were provided for the county boroughs in 1878. The county medical officer of health was an officer of the county council and was made responsible for the efficient operation of the tuberculosis service and the school medical service administered by the council. He was, however, also responsible for the infectious diseases services, the maternity and child welfare services and the other preventive services which came under boards of health and public assistance in rural areas and urban district councils in urban districts. Through the county medical officer of health, co-ordination could be effected among these services, but his responsibilities did not extend to the dispensary medical service, the general hospital service or the care of the mentally ill.

These arrangements for local administration lasted until 1942, when they were substantially altered by the introduction of the county management system. The management system, under which a salaried manager took over responsibility for the day-to-day executive functions of the elected members of a local body, had been introduced earlier for the corporations of Dublin, Cork, Limerick and Waterford. By the County Management Act, 1940, it was extended to all areas. As a corollary of this step, the boards of health and public assistance were abolished, their work being taken over by the county councils and the managers. The urban district councils remained, but the county manager acted for them as well as for the county council.

The significance of these changes lay in that the county managers took over all the detailed administrative work and much of the formulation of local policy on all the health services. However, the law still recognised the distinction between public assistance authorities, sanitary authorities and mental hospital authorities, and the three divisions of the services were not at this point integrated to any significant extent. Nevertheless, the alterations made by the introduction of county management set the stage for some fundamental re-thinking on several aspects of the services and their administration.

Finance

The basis for financing the services remained unchanged during this period. The local rates continued to meet most of the cost, but for some services rather more generous state assistance was provided. Special grants were introduced to meet half of the cost of the tuberculosis service, the school medical service and the maternity and child welfare schemes, and a similar grant met three-quarters of the expenditure on venereal diseases schemes. Finally, in 1932, a fixed amount grant, was introduced to finance the provision by local authorities of free milk to necessitous children. As described above, the Hospitals Trust Fund became an important new source of moneys for the health services, in the nineteen-thirties.

Personnel

After the creation[5] in 1908 of the National University of Ireland and its three constituent colleges in Cork, Dublin and Galway, medical schools became established in these colleges, assimulating schools already in existence to meet primarily the needs of the Catholic population. These schools were recognised under the Medical Act, 1858, for the inclusion of graduates in the United Kingdom register. In 1927, a

27

separate Irish medical register was established under a new statutory body, the Medical Registration Council.[6] Another body, the Dental Board, was set up in 1928 to govern the dental profession and, in conjunction with the Medical Registration Council, the training of dentists. Midwifery was controlled under an act passed in 1918. This established a board to register qualified midwives and to prevent unqualified persons from practising. In 1919, the training and qualification of nurses came under the General Nursing Council of Ireland. The formal structures for the health professions thus became firmly established and the levels of training were being constantly enhanced. As far as the local authority services were concerned, the selection of senior personnel was very significantly improved when it was transferred to the Local Appointments Commission[8] in 1926. Selection by the commission through impartial interview boards replaced election by vote of the local authority members (often bought) in the choice of dispensary doctors, county surgeons and other senior professional personnel.

ASSESSMENT OF THE PERIOD 1900–1945

Structurally, the health services benefited from the legislative and administrative changes made in this period. However, war and economic depression prevented any fundamental reformation of services or the provision of major extra public finance for them (the most costly development—the building of the county hospitals—would probably not have gone ahead in the absence of the sweepstakes). The most significant changes were on the preventive side. The county medical officers of health, as they developed the school medical service, the schemes for maternity and child care, the tuberculosis service and the general infectious diseases service, uncovered widespread health problems. Their reports to the local authorities and reports from other sources identified the extent of preventible illness and ill health in the community. In 1940, the expectation of life at birth in Ireland was 59 years for males and 61 for females, the death rate was 15 per 1,000 population and the infant mortality rate 75 per 1,000 live births, all rates in the ranges experienced at the present time in Third World countries. While little was possible before the war ended in 1945 to improve the services or to introduce new services to meet the needs that had thus become clear, thought was evolving on radical changes in the services.

NOTES ON CHAPTER TWO

1. Ruth Barrington, *Health, Medicine and Politics in Ireland, 1900-1970,* Dublin, Institute of Public Administration, 1987, page 39 et seq.
2. Under the Public Health (Prevention and Treatment of Disease) (Ireland) Act, 1918.
3. Barrington, op cit, page 93.
4. Under the Local Government Act, 1925.
5. Under the Irish Universities Act, 1908.
6. Under the Medical Practitioners Act, 1927.
7. Under the Dentists Act, 1928.
8. Established under the Local Authorities (Officers and Employees) Act, 1926.

CHAPTER THREE

1945–1965

The fruits of the thinking of the preceding years were to appear in 1945 and the following years. Mr Sean MacEntee had become Minister for Local Government and Public Health in 1942 in the Fianna Fail government. His parliamentary secretary on the health side was the long-serving Dr Con Ward.

The first fruits were the Tuberculosis (Establishment of Sanatoria) Act, 1945, which allowed the department itself to build new hospitals for the care of tuberculosis patients, and the Mental Treatment Act, 1945 referred to in the preceding chapter. These were non-contentious, but this was not the case with another bill introduced at the time – the Public Health Bill, 1945. This bill proposed many changes (some drastic) in the laws on the control of infectious diseases, on food hygiene and on similar preventive measures but the part which was to give rise to most opposition was that intended to provide for a wide extension of maternity and child care services without a means test, including general practitioner services for children up to sixteen years of age. It fell to Dr Ward to steer the bill through the Dail against vehement opposition. He had almost managed this when he left office in July 1946. The Public Health Bill was then put aside temporarily.

In the meantime another bill, the Ministers and Secretaries (Amendment) Bill, 1946, had been prepared. It's objective was the establishment of two new departments – for health

30

and for social welfare. It was passed in the autumn and the Department of Health was duly set up in January, 1947. The first Minister for Health was Dr James Ryan. He re-introduced Dr Ward's bill (with some changes) and it became law as the Health Act, 1947, in August. It was followed in 1947 by another act designed to give much more generous financial aid from the state for the development of the health services by the local authorities.

Two general schemes for the reform of the health system had been put on the table by this time. One was prepared in 1945 by Dr John Dignan, Bishop of Clonfert, who was chairman of the National Health Insurance Society.[1] It proposed a complete restructuring of the existing services, with an extension of eligibility, the financing of the services from an expanded scheme of insurance contributions and the transfer of their administration from the local authorities to the insurance system. The other scheme was put forward by the Irish Medical Association.[2] It proposed a scheme of health insurance for the middle class and retention of the dispensary system for the class entitled to it at the time. Neither scheme evoked a positive response from the minister.

The further plans of the government for the improvement of the health services were contained in a white paper issued in September, 1947.[3] This postulated an extension of hospital services to most of the population and general practitioner services, based on the dispensary system, to considerably more than were covered by it at the time. This was expressed to be an interim policy: the long term objective was 'a health service available to all citizens free of charge'. The white paper stimulated the medical profession to prepare for a fight against the changes proposed. In the meantime the Catholic Hierarchy had written to the government expressing objections to some of the provisions in the 1947 Health Act. Dr Ryan had not got the opportunity to use his formidable negotiating skills to attempt to overcome the objections of either of these two parties before he lost office with the change of government in February 1948.

The Minister for Health in the inter-party government

which took office then was Dr Noël Browne. He became minister on his first day in the Dail and was determined to push ahead fast with the development of the services – especially the tuberculosis service. He was fortunate in that no new legislation was needed for what he wanted to do. The 1945 Act had provided for the building of the regional sanatoria and preparatory work had started. The 1947 Health Act had made it clear that treatment in sanatoria would be free for all, had provided for a scheme of maintenance allowances for dependants of persons undergoing treatment, had made all cases of tuberculosis notifiable to the county and city medical officers and had made provision for a rehabilitation service designed for the needs of those recovered from the disease. The new arrangements for grants to the local authorities had removed any grounds for objection by them at that time to the developments because of an effect on the rates. Neither was finance a serious obstacle for capital schemes as money was again flowing into the Hospitals Trust Fund from the sweepstakes, which had been re-commenced after the war. Thus, the scene was set for the new minister to go ahead with the developments which he wanted. The tide was flowing with him.

Dr Browne's drive and enthusiasm spurred the department and the local authorities to achieve his aims in combating tuberculosis within a timescale which many thought would be impossible. New beds were made available by converting some hospitals and other buildings to sanatoria, chest surgery centres were established, vaccination against the disease was introduced and a mobile mass x-ray service developed. New drugs to treat the disease were used as they became available. Within three years the death-rate from tuberculosis had halved.

Part III of the Health Act, 1947, dealing with mother and child services, remained dormant until June 1950, when the minister circulated detailed proposals for implementing it. There was strong dissent from the medical profession and the Catholic Hierarchy voiced objections which they had to the scheme. Dr Browne failed to get the support of the government for proceeding with his scheme and resigned in April 1951. Three months later, the Dail was dissolved. In the meantime the Taoiseach, Mr John A. Costello, held the health portfolio. These events are referred to again in page 44 but in this thumbnail sketch any discussion on the actions and motivations of those involved in this controversy is out of the question. It is very well covered in Dr J.H. Whyte's *Church and State in Modern Ireland 1923-1970* [4] and in Dr Ruth Barrington's *Health, Medicine and Politics in Ireland, 1900 – 1970*.[5] Dr Browne's own story is given in his autobiography, *Against the Tide*.[6]

After the election in June 1951, Fianna Fail were back in power and Dr Ryan was again Minister for Health. A new white paper on the health services was issued in 1952.[7] This and the bill issued subsequently repeated the commitment to the development of a maternity and infant care scheme, and provided for child welfare clinic services and school health examinations and for some other new services. The 1947 proposal for general practitioner services for all children under sixteen was dropped but the new bill provided for the extension of eligibility for hospital services to about eighty-five per cent of the population.

During discussions on the white paper and on the bill which was to implement it, the minister made a number of changes to meet views expressed by the Hierarchy and the medical profession. Nevertheless the profession did not drop their opposition to the bill but Dr Ryan went ahead with it, under the impression that he had satisfied the Hierarchy. He had not: in April, they issued a statement to the press objecting to a number of provisions of the bill. Following an urgent meeting which the Taoiseach, Eamonn De Valera and the minister arranged with Cardinal D'Alton, the statement was withdrawn from the press. There were further discussions with the Hierarchy and agreement was reached on certain amendments. These were significant but did not alter the main purposes of the bill. It became law in October 1953.

Before the new act could be implemented, there was

another change of government and Dr Ryan was replaced as Minister for Health by Mr T.F.O'Higgins. While this act was not quite what he or his party, Fine Gael, would have sponsored from the start, the new inter-party government were committed to implementing it. The expanded hospital and maternity and child care services commenced in March 1956. The final significant piece of legislation in this period was the act, sponsored by Mr O'Higgins, which established the Voluntary Health Insurance Board in 1957.

Mr Sean MacEntee who, as Minister for Local Government and Public Health, had responsibility for health policies in the early nineteen-forties, become Minister for Health in the new Fianna Fail government in March 1957. The country was in a state of economic stagnation at the time. The government's policy, as expressed in the Programme for Economic Expansion published in 1958, was to give precedence in the allocation of resources to economic development. Hence, social services, including health, were put on a 'care and maintenance' basis during Mr MacEntee's term of office. He put through a programme of useful legislation, including the Health Authorities Act, 1960, the Health (Fluoridation of Water Supplies) Act, 1960, the Health (Corporate Bodies) Act, 1961 and the Health (Homes for Incapacitated Persons) Act, 1964. On the core issues of eligibility and the structuring of services, government policy did not, however, allow for substantial development at that time.

The Fine Gael and Labour parties had published their proposals for expansion (the former favoured a comprehensive health service financed largely by insurance contributions for eighty-five per cent of the population and the latter a service free of charge to all). When a motion in November 1961 by Deputy O'Higgins on his party's scheme raised the possibility of defeat for the government in the Dail, Mr MacEntee proposed the establishment of a select committee of the house to examine the health services and make recommendations. This proposal was agreed by the Dail. The committee was set up in 1961. It continued to meet until April 1965 when it ceased to exist with the dissolution of the Dail.

SERVICES 1945–1965

General hospital services
The liability of the local authorities to provide inpatient and outpatient hospital services was widely extended. Under the Health Act, 1953, eligibility was extended to a much broader class and became related not to individually-tested lack of means but to membership of one or other of four classes—persons insured for social welfare, persons with family incomes less than £600 a year, farmers with farms valued at or under £50 and those outside these groups who could demonstrate 'undue hardship'.[8] Some of these were entitled to the services without charge; statutory charges (originally six, later ten, shillings a day) were fixed for others and higher charges could be made for some of those brought in as hardship cases. Eligibility for out-patient specialist services was governed in a similar way.

With the development of these services, the similar facilities for insured workers under the 'additional benefits' scheme of the Department of Social Welfare described on page 24 were withdrawn. The development of the new service, particularly in the Dublin area, involved an increased acceptance by local authorities of responsibility for the cost of treatment of patients in voluntary hospitals. The income limit of £600 was raised to £800 in 1958, to make allowance for the fall in the value of money since 1953. This and subsequent adjustments were designed to retain the eligibility level for the services at about 85 per cent of the population.

This extension of eligibility was accompanied by a widespread extension of hospital facilities. The post-war hospital building programme had provided for the reconstruction or extension of 128 hospitals, sufficient to meet the new demands. Many extra consultant and other posts had been created in the regional and county hospitals.

The mentally-ill and the mentally handicapped
The introduction of the procedures for admission to and discharge from psychiatric hospitals introduced by the 1945

Act was timely. Better understanding of the nature of mental illness and the development of new therapies in the nineteen-fifties, particularly the use of anti-depressants and other psychotropic drugs, made it easier to contemplate alternatives to institutional care. The number of patients in the psychiatric hospitals began to fall in 1958, when it had reached its maximum of about 21,000. The development of out-patient clinics, some at general hospitals, commenced in this period. The extension of entitlement to general hospital services introduced in 1953 was matched by a corresponding extension for the psychiatric hospitals.

The county homes
As mentioned on page 20, some of the workhouses had become county homes for the able-bodied poor under the schemes drawn up in the early nineteen-twenties. Far-reaching changes were envisaged at that time (mainly by way of better segregation of inmates) but, except in a few areas, little was done. No aid was given from state funds towards capital costs or running expenditure on the homes. In 1951, an interdepartmental committee reported on the county homes and found that the conditions in many of them were unsatisfactory. They recommended that the homes should cater only for the aged and the chronic sick and that others in them (such as the mentally handicapped) should be accommodated elsewhere. A white paper based on this report[9] indicated government acceptance of the committee's recommendations. The local authorities were asked to act on them and, to encourage them to do this, a state grant to meet half of the cost of loan changes on capital expenditure for the improvement of the homes was introduced.

The dispensary medical service
No fundamental changes were made in the dispensary service during this period. There was, however, an improvement in the arrangements for deciding on eligibility. The issue of 'red tickets' each time a person needed care was dropped in favour of annual 'medical cards' issued by the health

36

authorities. However, there were wide and inexplicable differences between the local authorities in the criteria used for assessing eligibility. The highest percentages of population covered on 31 December 1958 were in Limerick City (54%) and Kilkenny County (46%) while the lowest were Dublin City and County (16%) and Leitrim County (20%).

The condition of the dispensaries had given rise to much criticism. As an example, Bishop Dignan in 1945 had stated:

> The dispensary is the core, the hub and heart of the degrading Poor Law system. To understand the system you have only to visit a dispensary. Most of them have no proper accommodation, no sanitary arrangements, no waiting rooms and, from the medical point of view, few conveniences and appliances to help the doctor to diagnose or to treat.[10]

To raise the standards of the dispensaries, a scheme of special grants for replacements built to a common design was introduced by the department in 1952. This scheme operated for five years during which 219 replacement dispensaries were built, about one-third of the total number.

Preventive services
The laws on the control of infectious diseases and on food hygiene, which dated back to the Public Health (Ireland) Act, 1878, were codified and modernised under the Health Act, 1947. The main innovations in this code were that free hospital treatment for infectious diseases became clearly available to all. The regulations to prevent the spread of infectious diseases from foreign-going ships were brought up to date and similar new regulations were introduced in relation to air traffic. The codification also involved the replacement of the provisions in the 1878 act for the prevention of the sale of diseased or unsound food by the Food Hygiene Regulations, 1950. These new provisions are described in chapter six.

Maternity and child care

The maternity and child care services prior to 1953 comprised attendance by dispensary medical officers and midwives on poor patients (with hospital care for them if necessary) and clinics and nursing services provided by health authorities or voluntary agencies in some areas. These services were considerably extended under the Health Act, 1953. Women in (or dependent on persons in) the four groups eligible for hospital services became entitled to a full maternity service, with choice of doctor and midwife and, on paying a contribution, choice of hospital or maternity home. Comprehensive medical and nursing care for their infants was also provided for. Maternity cash grants of £4 for each birth were introduced for women in what became known as the lower income group. A requirement on health authorities to provide child welfare clinic services was substituted for the permission to do so which was given to them under earlier law and new regulations were made for the improvement of the school health services.

General policy on health care

The policy which evolved from this period and to which concrete expression was given in the Health Act, 1953, can be summarised as providing for each class the services which the persons in it could not themselves afford. Thus, the general practitioner service remained available only to those who could individually demonstrate need, and the institutional services, being more costly, were provided for a wider group. Apart from the extension of the latter services to a greater proportion of the population, the main change in them lay in the statutory specification of the general groups eligible, in place of the previous individual assessment of need. A broad-spectrum means test replaced the unpalatable assistance basis of the earlier services. Once a person could show that he was in one of the statutory groups, his entitlement became independent of an official's judgement on his need for the service.

Section 4 of the Health Act, 1953, set out a principle

underlying the provision of services under the act. It reads:

(1) Nothing in this Act or any instrument thereunder shall be construed as imposing an obligation on any person to avail himself of any service provided under this Act or to submit himself or any person for whom he is responsible to health examination or treatment.

(2) Any person who avails himself of any service provided under this Act shall not be under any obligation to submit himself or any person for whom he is responsible to a health examination or treatment which is contrary to the teaching of his religion.

This section still remains in force.

ADMINISTRATION

Central administration
The establishment of the separate Department of Health is referred to on page 31. The combination of local government and health in one department had brought a large number of wide-ranging services under one minister. Many of these, not only on the health side, stood in need of review after the war and, to permit adequate attention to be given to the impending changes in the health services, the separate department was established.

The functions of the Department of Health were defined in the 1947 White Paper as including 'the administration and business relating to the preparation, effective carrying out and co-ordination of measures conducive to the health of the people, including in particular measures for:

the prevention and cure of disease;

the treatment and care of persons suffering from physical defects or mental illnesses;

the regulation and control of the training and registration of persons for health services;

control over the appointment and conditions of service of appropriate local officers;

the initiation and direction of research;

ensuring that impure or contaminated food is not marketed and that adequate nutritive standards obtain in essential foodstuffs;

the control of proprietary medical and toilet preparations;

the registration of births, deaths and marriages;

the collection, preparation, publication and dissemination of information and statistics relating to health.

Responsibility for the water supplies, sewage disposal and other sanitary services remained with the Department of Local Government, it being agreed that the Department of Health would provide advice on the medical questions arising in the provision of these services.

A distinctive feature in the development of central administration in the period after 1945 was the extent to which consultative bodies, representative of vocational and other interests, were established to advise the Minister for Health. The most important of these was the National Health Council. This council was first established under the Health Act, 1947. The minister, in constituting it, included nominees of a number of professional organisations but there was no obligation on him to do so. The council met only when called together by the minister and had authority to advise him only on subjects nominated by him. The council's status was improved under the Health Act, 1953, when it was given authority, within limits, to meet of its own volition and to advise the minister on subjects of its own choice; the 1953 act also provided that at least half of the members be nominated by bodies representing the medical and ancillary professions and persons concerned with the management of voluntary hospitals. A number of specialist consultative councils were also appointed in this period.

Local administration

As described above the development of the local government system had resulted in a number of different types of local authorities being concerned with the administration of health services. The trend in this period was towards a reduction in the numbers and types of authorities and towards the abolition of legal distinctions between different branches of the services. The first steps in this direction were taken under the Health Act, 1947. The simplification achieved under that act was mainly in the transfer of responsibility for the preventive services in the urban districts (apart from the county boroughs) to the county councils. This meant that for diphtheria immunisation, infectious disease control, food hygiene and some other services, the number of responsible authorities was reduced from about ninety to thirty-one. As the county councils were also the public assistance authorities in most areas, the change made by this act meant that in most areas one body was administering most of the health services.

The legal distinction between the services under the Health Acts and those administered by public assistance authorities remained until responsibility for the latter services was transferred to the health authorities under the Health Act, 1953. Under that act, the county and district hospitals which, as 'district institutions', were providing care under the public assistance authorities for 'poor persons unable by their own industry or other lawful means' to provide such care for themselves, joined the sanatoria in the category of 'health institutions', under the health authorities. The county council was both health authority and public assistance authority in most areas. This may not appear an important change, but it opened the way for more flexibility in the use of institutions.

This change in the legal status of the hospitals cleared the path for a definite break with the old poor law tradition in the administration of these institutions. Up to 1954, the regulations[11] governing county homes and county and district hospitals were redolent of the poor law. These regulations stated, for example, that 'a person admitted as an inmate

41

shall, if circumstances so require and permit, before being placed in the appropriate part of the institution, be thoroughly cleansed, unless the medical officer of the institution otherwise directs, and be suitably clothed', that a person on admission might 'be searched for intoxicating liquor or other article, the introduction of which is prohibited by the public assistance authority', and that, as a concession, an 'inmate' might, 'if the matron or head nurse so approved, be permitted ...... to wear or use any clothing or other articles belonging to him'. Whatever dubious reasons there might have been for such provisions in earlier times, clearly they had to go when the services in these hospitals were being made available to wider groups under the act of 1953.

New local consultative health committees, including medical representatives, were set up under the Health Act, 1953. Their function was to advise the city and county managers on the operation of the general health services.

The net effect of the changes in the law on local administration under the Health Acts of 1947 and 1953, was that the county council, as health authority, administered all the health services, except for the mental treatment service, in most parts of the country. The administration of mental hospitals was still governed by a separate code (the Mental Treatment Act, 1945) and was in most areas in the hands of special joint boards.

In the Dublin, Cork, Limerick and Waterford areas, there remained complexes of health authorities, public assistance boards and mental hospital boards until, under the Health Authorities Act, 1960, there was established in each of these areas a unified authority with comprehensive responsibility for all the health services. These four unified health authorities were joint bodies within the local government system, the entire membership in each case being made up of local councillors nominated by the county and city council involved (and, in the case of the Dublin Health Authority, the Dun Laoghaire Borough Council).

By 1960, the number of the local authorities responsible for the health services had thus been reduced to twenty-seven (these four unified authorities and the county councils elsewhere). This was the culmination of the long trend towards having bigger and fewer local authorities responsible for health care: no further development within the local government system was to take place.

Finance
We have seen that in earlier periods the local rates, supplemented by modest state grants, were called upon to bear the cost of the health services. In 1947, the grants totalled about £830,000 and met sixteen per cent of the cost of the services. When, after the war, plans were prepared for substantial developments and extensions of the services, it was clear that more generous financial assistance from the state would be needed. The 1947 white paper indicated that state subvention towards the cost would be substantially increased over the following years. Effect was given to this promise by the Health Services (Financial Provisions) Act, 1947. The basic principle of this act was simple. The state undertook to meet, for each health authority, the full amount of any increase in the cost of its services until the total cost was twice the amount met by that authority from local taxation in the year to 31 March 1948. When the cost of the services rose above that level, it was to be divided equally between the rates and the Exchequer. In other words, the state paid for all the increases until it was paying as much as the local authority and thereafter it met half of any increase. The object was to remove or reduce any financial grounds for lack of local enthusiasm for the development of the services.

Voluntary health insurance
The statutory health services offered little at this time to those in the upper income group (estimated to constitute about 15 per cent of the population). An advisory body was set up by the minister, Tom O'Higgins, in 1956 to examine the feasibility of a state-sponsored voluntary health insurance scheme to meet the needs of this group. Arising out of the

report of this body, a bill was introduced which became the Voluntary Health Insurance Act, 1957. This act set up a board to operate voluntary health insurance schemes, mainly for hospital care, on a non-profit-making basis. The public response was good. By the end of 1958, the board's various schemes covered a total of some 57,000 people and the numbers covered continued to grow in the following years.

ASSESSMENT OF THE PERIOD 1945–1965

The changes in this period – particularly its first decade – were of a different order of magnitude from any in earlier years. The role of the state in health care, which had been largely in prevention, was extended to cover the organisation and financing of curative medicine for wide groups of the population. The separate Department of Health was set up and the scale of state finance was increased to pay half of the cost of running the services. While the services were still largely within the local government system, the part of that system managing them was streamlined.

As mentioned earlier, these changes – especially the widening of the scope of services – cut across existing interests, particularly the medical profession and the Catholic Hierarchy. To meet points made by the Hierarchy, the state agreed to include safeguards in its legislation. The medical profession was slower in coming to realise that it had to live with state medicine on a large scale but eventually it did.

For its part, the Department of Health thereafter established generally satisfactory working relations with the medical profession (and the other health professions). It came to recognise the value of flexibility and the need to communicate its proposals accurately (the phrase 'education of women in respect of motherhood' in the 1947 Health Act had conveyed to some a meaning going outside the health field which had not been in the minds of those who wrote it).

On the 'mother and child' scheme, one must remember

that it contained two elements – firstly, the health care of mothers and infants (which did come into operation) and secondly, the proposal for general practitioner services without means test for all children up to sixteen years of age (which was dropped in 1952). The basis for this part of the scheme was to have been the dispensary system (albeit upgraded), with the district medical officers in a hierarchal relationship with the county medical officers. Had this been pushed through in that form, it is doubtful if it would have survived for long. If it had, it could have been at the expense of the greater priority of the period, which lay in the extension of eligibility for hospital services.

Looking back, one can say that the mother and child controversy served a good purpose in forcing re-thinking on priorities and in opening minds.

Ruth Barrington comments as follows:

> Perhaps those who gained most from the controversies of these years were the ordinary Irish people, whose chances of dying from an infectious disease in infancy, or tuberculosis in adulthood, of complications in childbirth or of suffering throughout life from disabling but treatable diseases, were greatly reduced. They now benefited from a health service of an incomparably higher standard than in the 1940s; and the extension of eligibility and provision of publicly guaranteed insurance had removed the fear of crippling medical costs. It was an achievement about which politicians, health administrators, doctors, and even bishops could be proud.[12]

Statistics support what she wrote. In 1961, the expectation of life for a male infant was 68 years and for a female 72. The infant mortality rate then was 30 per 1,000 live births. No longer could one describe Ireland's health status as being of the Third World.

NOTES ON CHAPTER THREE

1. J. Dignan, Bishop of Clonfert: Social Security, Outlines of a Scheme for National Health Insurance, Sligo, 1945.
2. Journal of Irish Medical Association, Vol 15, No. 90, Dec. 1944.
3. White Paper: Outline of Proposals for the Improvement of the Health Services, 1947 (P. No. 8400)
4. J. H. Whyte, *Church and State in Modern Ireland*, 1923-1970, Gill and Macmillan, 1971.
5. R. Barrington, *Health Medicine & Politics in Ireland 1900-1970* Institute of Public Administration, 1987.
6. N. Browne, *Against the Tide,* Gill and Macmillan, 1986.
7. White Paper: Proposals for Improved and Extended Health Services, 1952 (Pr 1333).
8. Health Act, 1953, section 15.
9. White Paper: Reconstruction and Improvement of County Homes, 1951 (Pr 756).
10. J. Dignan, op cit.
11. Public Assistance (General Regulations) Order, 1942 (SR&O No 83 of 1942).
12. Barrington, op cit, page 250.

CHAPTER FOUR

1965-1987

The nineteen-sixties was a period of scrutiny of existing services, of identification of problems, and of recommendations – sometimes contradictory – for solutions. It was a period of uncertainty for some existing services pending decisions on changes. It was a period of new medical discoveries and of a change in emphasis in the aims of the health services, because of the decline in some former problems, the intensification of others and the emergence of some new ones. Heart disease, cancer, psychiatric conditions (including those associated with alcoholism and drug dependence), diseases connected with ageing and accidents emerged as the main concerns for the seventies and eighties. Just as was the case with tuberculosis in earlier times, these were problems rooted in the way of life of the people, but because the way of life had become so much more complex, solutions to these problems were clearly going to be much more difficult to find.

These years saw a realisation and acceptance of the fact that the new fruits of medical science could not easily be made available to all who could benefit from them and that, because of the complexity of modern medical organisation, changes and new involvements in health administration were called for. This was a period too within which the awesome nature of the financial problem of the health services became evident, not only in this country. The need for ordered priorities in health expenditure became more apparent.

During the campaign before the general election in April

1965, the Taoiseach, Mr Sean Lemass, announced that Fianna Fail, if returned to power, would continue to improve the health services and that the next development would be the introduction of a choice of doctor in the general medical service. His party did again form the government and a new Minister for Health was appointed, Mr Donogh O'Malley. He was given a brief to fulfill the promise made by the Taoiseach. Clearly the tide had turned for the health services.

The Dail Select Committee on the Health Services had not issued a report but, during the years of its existence, it had gathered written submissions from a wide range of interests and had heard oral evidence from some. The Department of Health had been involved in analysing issues raised and in identifying options for change. The new minister had been a member of the committee (as had his predecessors, Messrs MacEntee and O'Higgins). Hence, the time was ripe for decisions on changes. Shortly after being appointed, Mr O'Malley initiated the preparation of a white paper on the development of the services. This was published in January, 1966[1]and formed the basis for most of the changes made in the following years. Donogh O'Malley did not remain long as Minister for Health: in July 1966, he was transferred to Education. It fell to Mr Sean Flanagan, his successor as Minister for Health, to continue the preparations for the changes announced in the white paper.

The main changes proposed were the introduction of a 'choice-of- doctor' scheme in place of the dispensary service, the transfer of the administration of the services from the local authorities to new health boards and the further augmentation of state finance for the services. There were reservations from different quarters on each of these. The new minister himself, having a rural background, was uneasy about the effect which the changeover to a 'choice-of-doctor' scheme might have in rural areas and this unease was shared by some local authorities and some elements of the medical profession. The proposed change in administration was, not unexpectedly, opposed by the local authorities and the Department of Finance did not look kindly on the prospect of the State paying a bigger share of the cost of the services.

Understandably, there was much consultation and study before the changes were put into the form of detailed proposals for legislation. Eventually, the proposals saw legislative form in the Health Bill, 1969. It had the distinction of being introduced at the special session commemorating the fiftieth anniversary of the First Dail, which was held in the Mansion House, Dublin in January 1969. The bill received a second reading in May but its course was then interrupted by the general election in July. Mr Erskine Childers was the Minister for Health in the new Dail. An experienced and assiduous parliamentarian, he applied himself to steering the Health Bill through the Oireachtas (it became law in February 1970) and to the follow-up work needed to bring it into operation. The far-reaching changes which were made are described and discussed later in this chapter and in other chapters. Erskine Childers had also given much attention to the restructuring of the hospital system. He lost office in March 1973 and was elected President of Ireland soon after.

In the new government, a coalition of Fine Gael and Labour, Mr Brendan Corish became Minister for Health. He was Tanaiste and head of the Labour Party and was also Minister for Social Welfare. He ran into trouble with the medical profession early in his ministry, when the first ever strike by junior hospital doctors arose out of long-smouldering grievances, and again in 1974, when he attempted to make a change in eligibility for hospital services so as to cover the entire population. He backed down when threatened with industrial action by hospital consultants. His main achievement as minister was to work out with the health boards a hospital plan under which the number of county hospitals giving full medical and surgical care would, over time, be reduced from twenty-four to fourteen, these fourteen to be expanded and developed so as to provide a better service in each area. Brendan Corish was also responsible for setting up the Health Education Bureau in 1975 and for the Misuse of Drugs Act, 1977 – a timely measure in the light of the explosion of the drug problem in the following years.

The tenth Minister for Health, Mr Charles Haughey, took up office in July 1977. He took advantage of a government policy of increased public spending to initiate many capital projects and additions to staff and other facilities. He concentrated on measures to prevent disease and encourage good health — notably the Tobacco Products (Control of Advertising, Sponsorship and Sales Promotion) Act, 1978. In April 1979, he arranged, in an entirely pragmatic way, an extension of hospital services (and some other services) to all income groups when the upper income limit for liability to pay health contributions was removed. To get over opposition from the medical profession, he allowed consultants to continue to charge fees on the top fifteen per cent or so of the population, even when in public wards. As over 25 per cent was covered by voluntary health insurance at this time, there were few in the top fifteen per cent who would not opt for private care, so this concession to the consultants was of little practical significance. It did not, however, please the Irish Congress of Trade Unions, except for one of its members—the Medical Union. The Health (Family Planning) Act, was enacted in 1979.

When Charles Haughey was elected Taoiseach in December 1979, Dr Michael Woods became Minister for Health. Dark clouds had built up in the economy and retrenchment in social spending was to be the main feature of the nineteen-eighties. Hence, there was little scope for new initiatives. There was a succession of short reigns as minister— Dr Woods until July 1981, Mrs Eileen Desmond (Labour Party) until March 1982 and Dr Woods again until December 1982.

Mr Barry Desmond (Labour Party) became minister for the next four years. He sponsored a considerable amount of legislation, including the Dentists Act, 1985 and the Nurses Act, 1985, which replaced the existing statutes on these professions, and acts amending the Misuse of Drugs Act, 1977 and the Health (Family Planning) Act, 1979.[2]

When the Labour ministers withdrew from the government in January 1987, Mr John Boland took over as Minister for

Health. After the general election in March 1987, Dr Rory O'Hanlon was appointed Minister for Health in the new Fianna Fail government.

THE SERVICES IN THE PERIOD SINCE 1965

The general medical service
The origin and nature of the dispensary system has been described in previous chapters. The 1966 white paper assessed the service and proposed a radical change in the following terms:

41.   The dispensary system has many merits. It ensures that everywhere, even in the most remote western districts, there will normally be at least one highly qualified and experienced medical practitioner to provide services for the lower income group (and, incidentally, for the rest of the people through his private practice). It provides all needed drugs, medicines and appliances for those in that group at no cost to them and at a moderate cost to public funds. That there is now considerable advocacy for replacing this service by one of a different kind does not detract from the quality of the service itself, nor reflect in any way on the work of the dispensary doctors who, for over a century, have been the strong foundation of our health services for the lower income group. But, with all its advantages, the dispensary system had one feature which must lead to its re-appraisal in any broad review of the health services in the context of social development: that is, that one who uses the service is set apart from a person who arranges for private medical care, in that he attends at the dispensary and not the doctor's private surgery, and has no choice of doctor. In assessing broadly the merits of the dispensary system, this feature must be accepted as outweighing the system's advantages and, now that many projects of greater priority in the improvement of our services have been

completed or are well advanced, the time has come when it is possible to consider replacing this system by one more akin to what is arranged privately by those outside the lower income group.

42.   The Government propose, therefore, that the general practitioner service organised by the health authorities should be re-arranged so that those whose medical care is paid for by the health authorities will be able to get the same kind of service as others can now get through private arrangement. This proposal involves substituting for the dispensary service a service with the greatest practicable choice of doctor and the least practicable distinction between private patients and those availing themselves of the service.

The white paper also stated that, in the context of a scheme for a choice of doctor, it would be preferable if drugs were supplied through the retail chemists (or the doctors themselves where this was not practicable).

    The implementation of these proposals had to await the enactment of the Health Act, 1970 and the completion of negotiations with the medical and pharmaceutical organisations on the details of the arrangements, which were protracted. The new general medical service based on these proposals commenced in the Eastern Health Board area on 1 April 1972, and in the rest of the country on 1 October 1972. It is described in chapter seven.

Services in hospitals and homes

Hospitals were becoming increasingly complex organisations, offering a wider range of skills for the diagnosis and treatment of diseases. As these skills became more sophisticated and specialised, increasing emphasis was placed on effective planning of hospital services and the avoidance of duplication and unnecessarily prolonged stays in hospital. The Fitzgerald Report[3] emphasised these points and recommended solutions to the problems involving a concentration of specialised hospital services in fewer centres. These services are discussed in chapter eleven.

Psychiatric services
New drugs and new methods of treatment for the mentally ill changed the pattern of care dramatically. There was an increased emphasis on out-patient treatment and the proportion of patients in mental hospitals who entered voluntarily had increased substantially. There was a large increase in the accommodation for the mentally handicapped and the facilities for them were improved in many respects. In chapters nine and ten, these changes are described.

Care of the aged
There was an increased recognition of the problems of the aged and of the need to develop specialised services for them. A number of other government departments and agencies are involved in this and the responsibility for co-ordinating activities was assigned to the Minister for Health and his department. An inter-departmental committee reported in 1968.[4] It recommended emphasis on community care and for those cases where this was inappropriate, well-planned care in hospitals and homes, including small welfare homes. This report was the basis for subsequent policies. In 1971, the National Social Service Council was set up by the minister to co-ordinate the activities of voluntary agencies and public authorities. The 1970 Health Act provided for the establishment of home help services.[5] Registration by health authorities of homes in which old people are maintained for profit had been provided for in 1964.[6] These services are described in chapter eight.

Preventive services
Perhaps the most noteworthy development was in the fluoridation of water supplies. This measure to prevent dental caries was provided for in the Health (Fluoridation of Water Supplies) Act, 1960. After an interesting, long-drawn-out but unsuccessful effort to have this act declared unconstitutional

by the courts, it was progressively implemented throughout the country and piped public water supplies are now mainly flouridated. Another notable new preventive measure was the highly successful oral poliomyelitis vaccination campaign in 1965. Following on this campaign, poliomyelitis has been almost eliminated from the community.

The period also saw a widening realisation of the need for further measures to protect the public from danger in the sale and distribution of drugs and poisons. The Poisons Act, 1961, gave the minister wider powers to make regulations on this and the Misuse of Drugs Act, 1977, gave better powers to control the abuse of drugs of addiction. Plans for improvements in the child health services were pushed ahead, the aim being to replace the child welfare clinic schemes and the school health examination service with a comprehensive well-planned service offering surveillance from infancy to the conclusion of primary schooling.

In these years there was a heightened emphasis on positive measures in the field of prevention. Health education was given a more prominent role, particularly in relation to smoking, alcohol-related diseases and drugs. The Tobacco Products (Control of Advertising, Sponsorship and Sales Promotion) Act, 1978, gave the Minister for Health wide powers to restrict the promotion of tobacco products. The original regulations spelling out the controls under this act were considerably strengthened by Barry Desmond during his term of office as minister.[7]

Voluntary health insurance
The Voluntary Health Insurance Board flourished during this period. The number of persons covered by the board's schemes increased substantially, the scheme of benefits was made more flexible and otherwise improved. The activities of the board are discussed in chapter sixteen.

ADMINISTRATION

Central administration

The report of the Public Services Organisation Review Group (PSORG), issued in 1969,[8] dealt with the reorganisation of government departments generally. The essential recommendation of this report was that ministers should divest themselves of direct executive responsibility for services, so as to be free to concentrate on the general planning, organisation and review of them. The report recognised that organisational developments in the health services arising from the 1966 white paper had been in accordance with this recommendation and a restructuring of the Department of Health on the principles of the report was accomplished during the period.

Several bodies were set up under the Health (Corporate Bodies) Act, 1961 during the period. Among them were the Medico-Social Research Board, the National Drugs Advisory Board and the Health Education Bureau. Another act transferred former workhouse lands to the local authorities[9] and in 1971, the administration of the Central Mental Hospital at Dundrum was transferred from the Department of Health to the newly established Eastern Health Board.[10] Both of these moves were in accord with the general policy to have detailed executive work devolved from the department.

The minister's powers to set up specialised advisory bodies were widely used during this period. In addition, the National Health Council continued to exercise its function of examining and reporting on the services. In 1972, there was an important change for the hospital services in the establishment of Comhairle na nOspideal, the body to govern the creation of new consultant medical posts in hospitals and to advise generally on hospital services. These changes are described in later chapters.

Local administration

The local authority administration described earlier remained in control of the services until March 1971: new health boards set up under the Health Act, 1970, took over on that date. The idea of taking health administration away from the local authorities was not new. The 1947 White Paper tentatively put forward a proposal for special bodies directly responsible to the Minister for Health to administer the health services, with provision for regional co-ordination, but this proposal was not followed up at the time. The idea of special bodies for the administration of the health services surfaced again in the 1966 white paper, in which it was proposed that legislation should be introduced to transfer the services to regional boards whose membership would 'represent a partnership between local government, central government and the vocational organisations'.

One might ask why there was such a long gestation period for what might seem to be an obvious move, viz. to split locally what had been split centrally when health and local government were made into separate departments of state in 1947. The answer may be that there was a reluctance to take health administration away from the local government system because, whatever doubt there might have been about the effectiveness of the local authorities in the nineteen-forties, it was clear, once the county management system had settled down, that the county councils and other health authorities provided, within the confines of the counties, a good system of administration and one which should not be tampered with without very good reason. It is very clear from the 1966 white paper that the eventual decision to take health administration away from the local authorities was not lightly reached. The white paper stated:

126. Notwithstanding the strong case for changing the administration of the health services in this way the Government would not wish the change to be made if there were a danger that the transfer from them of their health functions would so diminish the scope of the local authorities' work that they would become ineffectual bodies evoking little interest in the community. This danger is not real. If the existing

local authorities lose the direct administration of the health services, which now makes up about one-third of their total activities, they will still remain, beneath the government itself, probably the most important administrative organs in the State. Shorn of their health functions, the county councils would but be restored, as respects the scope of their work, to what they were in the nineteen-thirties, as health services of our present-day scope are quite a recent addition to their functions. The local councils will retain responsibility for the general planning and development of their areas, for the improvement and maintenance of the roads system, for housing development, for sanitary services and for several other general local government functions. The local government services are all developing and it is, indeed, better that local councils and county managers should in future be able to give them their undivided attention.

The case for the change in health administration, as stated in the white paper, had two bases. The first was that, because the State had taken over the major financial interest in the health services and this interest was increasing, it was desirable that a new administrative framework combining national and local interests should be developed for the services. The second basis for a change arose from the developments in professional techniques and equipment, which meant that better services could be provided on an inter-county basis. This argument was, of course, of greater relevance in the hospital services. For many of these services, and for the general organisation of hospital services, the county had become too small as a unit. In 1966, over half of all in-patients in acute hospitals were being treated in the regional and teaching hospitals in the larger centres, and specialist services at out-patient departments were being organised increasingly on a regional basis. It had become clear that the future efficiency of the hospital services was becoming more and more dependent on full co-ordination of the various units and that a board covering a number of counties could plan and arrange the hospital services for those counties so as to serve better the people in its area. From many counties, hundreds of patients were being sent annually at the expense of the local health authority to hospitals in other areas, but in these circumstances, the county concerned had no say in the organisation or operation of these hospitals. The grouping of counties under new bodies, representative of all counties within the group, meant that each county could become directly associated with the hospital centres to which most of its patients were traditionally sent and have a voice in the creation of policy on the services in those centres.

Based on these arguments, the case was made for the organisation of the hospital services in larger units. The option was open to do this and to leave the other health services, such as the general practitioner service and the preventive services, with the local authorities. This option was, however, rejected because always in mind as the main consideration was the importance of unitary control and responsibility for all the health services in each area. The services are all interdependent. Hospital care is related to what general practitioners do and may be an alternative to general practitioner care, and, of course, the activities of the preventive services can also affect the requirements for hospital and other services. It was, therefore, decided that it would be an essential principle of the new administration that one body would be responsible for the operation of all the health services in its area.

It was, in any event, apparent that many of the health services outside hospitals — such as general practitioner services, public health nursing services and child welfare services — would benefit from being organised across county boundaries. Many of our cities and towns straddle such boundaries (examples are Limerick, Waterford, Ballinasloe, Clonmel, Drogheda, Carrick-on-Suir and New Ross). With inter-county administration, such towns can be used more effectively as bases for these services. It was apparent too that larger units of administration would allow for the more economic employment of social workers and other staff for the child care and geriatric services.

The impact of the Fitzgerald Report

The publication in June 1968, of the Fitzgerald Report[3] influenced further thinking on these proposals. This report was concerned mainly with the sizes and kinds of hospitals needed to meet modern requirements, but it also made recommendations on administration, which would have left the control of hospital services separate from that of the other health services. It recommended an administrative system for the hospitals with a central body to control the distribution of specialities and the allocation of consultants, with three regional hospital boards based on the medical teaching centres of Dublin, Cork and Galway (in which hospitals would be vested) and with special management committees for individual hospitals or groups of hospitals. For the reasons outlined above, this separate system of administration did not commend itself, but it was accepted that special co-ordinating bodies would be desirable for the hospital services. It was accordingly decided to set up three regional hospital boards based on the medical teaching centres and with functions 'in relation to the general organisation and development of hospital services in an efficient and satisfactory manner in the hospitals administered by health boards and other bodies in its functional area which are engaged in the provision of services under the Health Acts.' These bodies did not find a satisfactory role in the structure and they are now defunct.

The Health Act 1970

The Health Bill, 1969 included provisions for setting up the health boards and the regional hospital boards and for the dissolution of bodies which would become redundant because of the changes, including the Dublin, Cork, Limerick and Waterford Health Authorities and the Hospitals Commission.

The provisions in the Health Act, 1970, for establishing

the new administrative system were broadly framed, leaving the details on the number and constitution of the health boards for subsequent regulations. However, so that the houses of the Oireachtas would later have an opportunity of approving or rejecting the detailed proposals, it was provided in the act that the regulations setting up the health boards would be subject to approval by resolutions of each house.

After discussion with the local authorities, the minister's proposals for the grouping of counties and the constitutions of the health boards were put into the form of draft regulations and these were approved by the Dail and Seanad. The regulations came into effect on 1 October 1970, so that the boards were legally established then. The process of appointing members was completed in November but they did not become responsible for the operation of the health services until 1 April 1971. The boards and their functional areas are described in chapter thirteen.

The 1970 act also provided for local committees to maintain contact at county level with the operation of the health services.

Finance
Up to 1966, the financial arrangements described in chapter three continued to apply. The Health Services Grant from the Exchequer met half of the cost of the services provided by the local authorities and the balance was met from local sources (the 'local sources', in fact, included some further state aid towards reducing the rates on agricultural land). A review of the existing financial system was included in the 1966 white paper. Having referred to the continuing trends towards increasing costs and having given estimates for the improvements and modifications in the services as then proposed, the white paper went on to state:

116.   *The Government, having studied this issue, are satisfied that the local rates are not a form of taxation suitable for collecting additional money on this scale. They propose, therefore, that the cost of the further extensions of the services should not be*

met in any proportion by the local rates. Following this decision, other possible sources of revenue to meet the additional costs are being considered but it seems likely that the general body of central taxation must bear the major part of the burden. *Pending further consideration of the methods by which extensions of the health services will be financed in future years, the Government have decided to make arrangements which will ensure that the total cost of the services falling on local rates in respect of the year 1966-67 will not exceed the cost in respect of the year 1965-66.*

The freeze on the rates contribution was not continued in full for succeeding years but grants supplementary to the statutory 50 per cent were paid so as to reduce the impact on the rates of the continuing rise in health expenditure. By 1970, the State grants specifically towards the health services were meeting 56 per cent of the total cost. The financial arrangements for the new health boards put these arrangements for supplementary grants on a formal basis.[11] In 1973, the government decided that the contribution from the rates to the cost of the health services would be phased out entirely. This move was completed by 1977.

Paragraph 116 of the white paper had referred to 'other possible sources of revenue' being considered. Among these sources was a scheme of contributions by eligible persons. Such a scheme was introduced in October 1971: it is described in chapter fifteen.

NOTES ON CHAPTER 4

1. White Paper: The Health Services and their Further Development, 1966 (Pr8653)
2. A full account of these years is contained in 'Report: Health Services, 1983–86' published by the Stationery Office, Dublin.
3. Outline of the Future Hospital System – Report of the Consultative Council on the General Hospital Services (Prl 154)
4. The Care of the Aged – Report of the Interdepartmental Committee, 1968(Prl 777)

5. Section 61
6. By the Health (Homes for Incapacitated Persons) Act, 1964
7. Under the Tobacco Products (Control of Advertising Sponsorship and Sales Promotion) Regulations, 1986
8. Report of Public Services Organisation Review Group, 1966 to 1969 (Prl 792)
9. The State Lands (Workhouses) Act, 1962
10. Under section 44 of the Health Act, 1970 and the Central Mental Hospital Order, 1971.
11. Section 32 of the Health Act, 1970.

CHAPTER FIVE

Eligibility for the services

The health services are for all the people but all the people
do not have access to all the services. What services an
individual is entitled to depends on his or her financial and
family circumstances. Earlier thinking on eligibility was
codified in the Health Act, 1970. This defined two groups,
those with 'full eligibility' and those with 'limited eligibility',
leaving a group of persons with higher incomes who were in
neither of these categories. The changes made in April 1979
extended 'limited eligibility' to include the last-mentioned
group. However, as will be seen below, some restrictions on
eligibility remained.

FULL ELIGIBILITY

Those with full eligibility are defined[1] as 'adult persons
unable without undue hardship to arrange general practitioner
medical and surgical services for themselves and their
dependants and dependants of such persons. It is stated that,
where a decision is taken as to whether or not a person
comes within this definition 'regard shall be had to the means
of the spouse (if any) of that person in addition to the
person's own means' (this removed a doubt in the
corresponding earlier definition which may have permitted
the incomes of other working members of the household to
be taken into account in taking similar decisions). The

criterion, therefore, as to whether a person has or has not full eligibility relates to his or her ability to pay for family doctor services. Apart from the clarification of the means to be taken into account, this is not much different from the earlier criterion of eligibility for the dispensary service.

The definition of full eligibility is relevant mainly to the general practitioner service which is described in chapter seven. The practical operation (and the economics) of this service are dependent on a clear definition of entitlement. Each health board, therefore, keeps a register of persons with full eligibility which it reviews periodically. Medical cards are issued to those in the register for presentation when services are needed.

These registers relate simply to entitlement to the general practitioner service, but the definition of 'full eligibility' is used for other services and purposes. In its interpretation for any particular service, there is a clause which permits the chief executive officer of the health board (or one of his subordinates) to exercise discretion and accept a hardship case as entitled.[2]

For some years, the chief executive officers of the eight health boards have agreed on guidelines for decisions on full eligibility which are applicable throughout the country. These are reviewed at intervals, usually annually. The guidelines in operation are set out in Appendix A. This also shows the numbers with full eligibility by county on 1 October 1987 and the general classification of those covered.

The decisions on which individuals have full eligibility are taken by officers of the health board (the board, as a body of members, are prohibited from intervening).[3] The primary decisions are taken locally by a subordinate officer and there is the right of appeal against refusal.

The Minister for Health has power to make regulations specifying 'a class or classes of persons who shall be deemed to be within the categories' having full eligibility.[4] Such regulations have not been made.

LIMITED ELIGIBILITY

When the concept of 'limited eligibility' was introduced,[5] those included within the concept were persons insured under the Social Welfare Acts (there was then an income limit for non-manual workers), other persons with yearly means under a fixed limit and farmers with valuations of £60 or less, and dependants of persons in each of these groups. There were complex requirements about social welfare contributions for non-manual workers.

The Health Services (Limited Eligibility) Regulations, 1979[6] replaced the complex definition in the 1970 act with a simple statement: 'A person who is without full eligibility shall have limited eligibility for services under this Part, (of the 1970 act)'. However, the Health Services Regulations, 1979 placed some restrictions on the 'limited eligibility' services available to the category with incomes at or above £5,500 a year. This limit has been reviewed from year to year. It currently stands at £15,000.

GENERAL PROVISIONS ON ELIGIBILITY

Health boards have power to require persons to make declarations in relation to means and to verify such declarations.[7] Where a person is recorded as entitled to a particular service, he is required to notify the board of any change in his circumstances which disentitles him to the service and if he obtains the service and it is found out that he was not entitled, he may be charged for it.[8] There are penalties also for false statements, etc., in relation to eligibility.[9]

CATEGORIES OF ELIGIBILITY

Because of the distinction in entitlement to services within the group with limited eligibility described above, it is more convenient to discuss entitlement to services by reference to the following three categories:

Category 1:
This category covers persons with full eligibility, as described above. Those in it are entitled to the full range of health services without charge. About 37 per cent of the population is in this category.

Category 2:
This covers persons, other than those in category 1, whose income in the preceding tax year is under the limit fixed, as mentioned above. The main benefits for them are hospital services (both maintenance and treatment) in public wards, specialist services in out-patient clinics and maternity and infant welfare services. About 45 per cent of the population is in this category.

Category 3:
The remainder of the population, that is persons whose income in the preceding tax year was above the fixed limit are in this category. They are entitled to in-patient and out-patient hospital services on the same basis as for those in category 2 except that they are liable to pay hospital consultants' fees. They are also entitled to other benefits as described below.

As regards categories 2 and 3, where a husband and wife have separate incomes, the eligibility of each is assessed separately. Where a dependent spouse has no income, he or she will be in the same category as the income-earner. The rule applicable to children under sixteen years of age is that, if both parents are in category 2, the children are included in that category but if either parent is in category 3, then the children are regarded as being in that category.

To distinguish between those in categories 2 and 3 for the purpose of hospital services, special arrangements are made by health boards. The object of this is to identify those in the former category on the basis of evidence of income in the preceding tax year (in most cases the Revenue Commissioners' form P60). It involves the issue of hospital services cards to those in category 2.

There are a number of services for which this division of the population is irrelevant. For example, treatment of infectious diseases is available free to all. Hospital treatment, both in-patient and out-patient is also available without charge for all children under sixteen years of age suffering from certain long-term ailments (see chapter eleven). Neither is there any means test for health examinations for pupils of national schools and health examinations at child health clinics or for out-patient specialist services for defects noticed at such examinations.

The table on page 68 shows, by category, the pattern of entitlement to the individual services.

NOTES ON CHAPTER FIVE

1. By section 45 of the Health Act, 1970. Adult persons are persons over sixteen years of age (see definition in section 2 of Health Act, 1947).
2. Section 45(7) of the Health Act, 1970
3. Section 17(3) and (4) of the Health Act, 1970
4. Section 45(3) of the Health Act, 1970
5. Under section 46 of the Health Act, 1970
6. Made under section 46(3) of the Health Act, 1970
7. Section 48 of the Health Act, 1970
8. Sections 49 and 50 of the Health Act, 1970
9. Section 75 of the Health Act, 1970

SERVICE	ENTITLEMENT
Community protection programme	
prevention of infectious diseases	all categories
child health examinations	all categories
other services (health education,	
drugs advisory service etc.)	all categories
Community health services programme	
general practitioner service	
(including prescribed drugs)	category 1
drug subsidy scheme	categories 2 and 3
scheme for drugs for long-term illnesses	categories 2 and 3
home nursing services	categories 1 and in some cases, categories 2 and 3
domiciliary maternity services	categories 1 and 2
family planning advisory service	all categories
dental, ophthalmic and aural services	
— for children	category 1 and, in some cases, categories 2 and 3
— for adults	category 1
Community welfare services	
schemes for cash payments, home helps, meals on wheels etc.	see pages 97 to 100
child care services	see pages 100 to 103
care of the aged	see page 103
Psychiatric programme	
service for diagnosis, care and prevention of psychiatric ailments	all categories—see page 106 for conditions
Programme for the handicapped	
care of mentally handicapped	all categories — see page 113 for conditions
care of blind, deaf and otherwise handicapped	all categories, see page 114 for conditions
rehabilitation service	all categories
General hospital programme	
services in public hospitals and subvention for patients in private hospitals	all categories, subject to charges for categories 2 and 3

This table does not demonstrate all the nuances of the conditions for eligibility. The chapters on the services give some more detail, but individual issues of eligibility can be determined only by the officers of the health boards.

CHAPTER SIX

Community protection programme

This chapter and the following two chapters deal with those health services which provide care outside hospitals and other institutions and with related welfare services. A series of programmes has beeen designed so that the community can enjoy a high level of personal health in a healthy environment. These are:

— the community protection programme (covering the prevention of infectious diseases, child health examinations, food hygiene and food standards, drug controls, health education and other preventive services);

— the community health services programme, covering general practitioner services (including the supply of drugs and medicines and schemes for subsidising drug purchases), home nursing services, domiciliary maternity services, family planning and dental, ophthalmic and aural services;

— the community welfare programme (including cash payments to disabled persons and to persons with certain infectious diseases, home helps and meals-on-wheels services, grants to voluntary welfare agencies, supply of free milk, maintenance of deprived children, welfare homes and other accommodation for the aged).

Earlier chapters have described how preventive health services were developed in conjunction with environmental protection by the local sanitary authorities, working first under the Local Government Board and later under the Department of Local Government and Public Health. Responsibility for this group of services at central level was split in 1947, when the Department of Health became responsible for the services relating to personal health and the Department of Local Government (now named the Department of the Environment) retained broad responsibility for services related to the environment. The division was made roughly between those services in which the medical content was predominant and those where engineering was the major factor. This split of responsibility is now reflected at local level where the health boards have taken over from the local authorities the responsibility for the personal health services but the environmental services have been left with the latter authorities. However, the medical officers of the health boards still advise the local authorities on medical aspects of housing, planning and development, water supplies, sewage disposal and other environmental problems.

CONTROL OF INFECTIOUS DISEASES

Communicable diseases no longer present problems of the same size as in earlier decades. Fortunately, the incidence of and the mortality rates from most of these diseases have declined so as to be almost negligible. The control of infectious diseases, for which the public health services were first organised, thus tends to pass into the background behind the new responsibilities of the health boards. This can be attributed to a number of factors, of which the more important are the development of vaccines and other prophylactic agents, improved sanitation and hygiene, new and improved drugs and the generally greater awareness within the community of the value of these preventive measures.

The infectious disease service, however, remains an important part of the community care programme and its continued smooth operation is essential if a re-emergence of major problems arising from infectious diseases is to be avoided or countered. The effectiveness of the service depends on notification, diagnosis and treatment (which is available without means test), prevention of the spread of infection, immunisation and vaccination, and the payment of maintenance allowances. There is a considerable body of law on these matters, mainly based on Part IV of the Health Act, 1947 and the regulations made under that part. The provisions of this body of law are summarised in Appendix B.

International travel
New problems were presented for the infectious disease service with the increase in international travel in recent decades. This trend, and in particular the rise in the numbers holidaying abroad each year, has called for greater organisation and greater alertness in the precautions necessary to safeguard the health of travellers and those with whom they come into contact. Responsibilities in this field rest mainly on those health boards whose areas include the major airports and seaports, but as most modern journeys, even from far-off countries, can be completed within the incubation periods of the most dangerous infectious diseases, all health boards must be watchful. Information leaflets are available to travellers, medical practitioners and travel agencies outlining the possible dangers to health when visiting other countries, particularly those with warm climates, and the precautions which should be taken by travellers.

Prophylaxis
The health boards' prophylactic campaigns have concentrated on diphtheria, poliomyelitis, whooping cough, rubella (german measles) and, more recently, measles. There were four immunisation schemes in operation in 1984. For diphtheria, 83% of the target group (children under two years of age) were immunised, for poliomyelitis 74% of the same group, for rubella 86% (girls 12 to 14 years) and for pertussis 43% (children under two years).[1]

71

Tuberculosis

Tuberculosis was probably the most feared disease in Ireland in the first half of this century. The incidence was severe and the death rate high (146 per 100,000 population in 1942). The disease attacked mainly the young and active and its tragic effects were often accentuated by its spread within families. This picture is now changed dramatically, as is illustrated in Table 1 below showing the trends in the incidence of the disease and in the death rate from it.

Table 1: *Tuberculosis*

	New cases notified	*Death rates per 100,000 population*
1952	6,685	60.0
1961	3,010	14.7
1971	1,238	6.1
1984	837	2.1

The downward trend in the death rate was interrupted in 1985, when there were 90 deaths, representing a rate of 2.5 per 100,000 population – indicating that the disease is not entirely conquered. There has been a marked shift in the incidence of the disease to the older age groups, particularly in the case of men.[2]

Other diseases

Of the other notifiable diseases, the most significant in numbers in 1985 were: measles 9,903 (6,180 in 1983), pertussis (whooping cough) 3,689 (1,728 in 1983), gastro-enteritis (in children under 5 years of age) 3,317 (2,987 in 1983), sexually transmissible diseases 2,869 (1984 figure; 2,567 in 1983), viral hepatitis 989 (1,482 in 1983), rubella (german measles) 668 (2,395 in 1983).[3]

AIDS

AIDS (acquired immune deficiency syndrome) is a condition in which the body's natural defence system has been attacked by a virus, the human immunodeficiency virus (HIV), and broken down so that this system cannot protect the body against infection and disease. This means that those with AIDS are at grave risk of infection and death from conditions which healthy people ordinarily overcome by their natural defence systems. AIDS has become a very serious problem in Central African countries and in the United States and cases have been reported from most European countries.

By January 1988, the Department of Health had been notified of thirty-one cases of full-blown AIDS in Ireland, of whom thirteen had died. There were indications, however, that about 700 persons were carrying the virus. The virus is spread from one person to another by intimate sexual contact or by exchange of blood (notably by sharing injection needles). To warn people whose way of life exposed them to the hazard of infection, the department and the Health Education Bureau launched a considerable publicity campaign.

SUPERVISION OF FOOD AND DRUGS

As part of their duties in controlling the spread of infectious diseases, health authorities have for long had functions in supervising the hygiene of food supplies. For the general well-being of the public, they have also had functions in relation to the quality and safety of food and drugs. Because our modern way of living is so dependent on processed and prepared foods and on an increasing variety of drugs and medicines, the efficacy of these controls is becoming increasingly important. Health boards now have a varied battery of legal powers to operate the controls in these fields.

Food hygiene

Hygiene in the manufacture, preparation, sale and serving of

73

food is governed by the Food Hygiene Regulations, 1950 to 1971. These regulations, together with the other legal provisions referred to in these paragraphs, are summarised in Appendix C and include a general prohibition of the sale of unfit food and give authority for the seizure of unfit food and power to stop the importation of such food. They also provide for the registration of food premises. The enforcement of the regulations is mainly in the hands of the health boards, acting through their medical officers and their health inspectors, who have special skills in this field.

Quality of food and drugs

The basic provisions on the general quality of food and drugs sold to the public are contained in the Sale of Food and Drugs Acts, 1875 to 1936. These were designed to prevent the sale of food or drugs which were injurious to health or 'not of the nature, substance or quality demanded by the purchaser.' Under these and later acts, there is also provision for fixing chemical standards for foods and power to make regulations controlling the use of preservatives, colouring matters and other additives. The enforcement of these provisions is mainly in the hands of the health inspectors.

Poisons and medical preparations

The sale and distribution of poisons and medical preparations are subject to a number of statutory controls. In 1982 regulations under the Poisons Act, 1961 replaced the earlier legislation on the control of poisons. Under that act, there is a statutory body, Comhairle na Nimheanna, to advise the minister on the regulations. Its members are mainly doctors and pharmacists. New regulations under the Health Act, 1947 have updated in 1987 earlier provisions on medical preparations and the Misuse of Drugs Acts, 1977 and 1984 have supplanted the Dangerous Drugs Act, 1934. The Control of Clinical Trials Act, 1987 gives powers to the minister relating to clinical trials of drugs and other substances. All these are described in Appendix C. This appendix also covers new regulations on cosmetics which implement directives of the European Community.

National Drugs Advisory Board
The National Drugs Advisory Board was established in July 1966[4] to provide a service to monitor newly-introduced medicinal products and to check their safety for human use. The board is also responsible for collecting and disseminating information on side-effects and reactions associated with drugs already in use, and for furnishing advice on precautions and restrictions in the marketing and use of such drugs. The board has sixteen members, appointed by the minister. The service provided by the board in relation to the assessment of drugs for safety was for a number of years a voluntary one, operated with the co-operation of the pharmaceutical industry. The introduction of a product authorisation scheme under the European Communities (Proprietary Medicinal Products) Regulations, 1974 and a scheme for the licensing of manufacturing and wholesale activities have placed these arrangements on a statutory basis. In 1985, the board's role was widened to cover the marketing of veterinary medicinal products.

Drug abuse
While, in the nineteen-sixties and seventies, there was concern over the abuse of drugs such as barbiturates and amphetamine, particularly by young people, a serious problem relating to the use of 'hard' drugs (in particular heroin) did not manifest itself in Ireland until the present decade. Following a report to the government by a special task force, the National Co-ordinating Committee on Drug Abuse was set up in March 1985 by the Minister for Health. It represents the various statutory and other bodies concerned with the drug problem.

It is naturally very difficult to gather precise figures on the extent of drug abuse. However, the following statistics of the numbers presenting for treatment at the National Drugs Advisory and Treatment Centre, Jervis Street, Dublin, the numbers of persons charged with drug offences, and the numbers of seizures of drugs give a good idea of the size of the problem.

Table 2: *Drug abuse*[5]

Year	Numbers presenting for treatment	Persons charged with drug offences	Drug seizures
1981	800	1,256	1,204
1982	1,307	1,593	1,873
1983	1,514	1,822	2,278
1984	1,454	1,369	1,704
1985	1,424	n.a.	n.a.

Heroin is the preponderant drug in these statistics.

The Jervis Street centre and the Coolmine Therapeutic Community, County Dublin, are the major special institutions for treatment of drug addicts. Facilities for the care and treatment of addicts are also available as part of the general services in psychiatric hospitals.[6] The health boards, and particularly the Eastern Health Board, are involved in local services for counselling and care.

The law on narcotic and similar dangerous drugs is contained in the Misuse of Drugs Acts, 1977 and 1984, which are described in Appendix C. The main objective of the 1984 act was to increase substantially the penalties for drug-related crimes, which now range up to life imprisonment for possession for unlawful sale or supply to others.

CONTROL ON TOBACCO PRODUCTS

Two reports published in the nineteen-sixties, by the surgeon-general in the United States and by the Royal College of Physicians in London, gave authoritative backing to conclusions reached by medical researchers that there were strong links between the consumption of tobacco (cigarette smoking in particular) and the incidence of a number of diseases notably lung cancer and heart disease. From this period on, health administrations throughout the world became active in campaigns to discourage the smoking habit by educating the public on its dangers and by controlling the promotional activities of the tobacco companies.

In Ireland the activities in this area were first based on discussions, aimed at voluntary curbs, with the trade and other interests. Some success was achieved but, by the nineteen-seventies, when further studies had confirmed the causative link between smoking and disease, it became clear that legislative powers were needed by the Minister for Health to control the promotion of tobacco products. Such powers were given in the Tobacco Products (Control of Advertising, Sponsorship and Sales Promotion) Act, 1978. This act gave the minister wide powers to make regulations defining and imposing such controls. The original regulations were made in 1979. These have since been superseded and strengthened by new regulations[7].

The effect of these regulations is:

to restrict the advertising media which may be used for tobacco advertising,

to limit the content of advertisements of tobacco products,

to require that advertisements for, and packages of, tobacco products display in rotation a number of prescribed health warnings,

to provide for the curtailment of expenditure on advertising and sponsorship,

to limit the form which advertising associated with sponsored events may take, and

to prohibit the use of coupons, gifts, cut-price offers and sales promotion in relation to tobacco products.

CHILD HEALTH EXAMINATIONS

As mentioned in earlier chapters, over a period of about fifty years, the local health authorities had developed a school health examination scheme for pupils of national schools and a child welfare clinic service. These services were examined by a study group appointed by the Minister for Health whose report was published in 1967.[8] The study group recommended that the existing services become a co-ordinated child health service and it made several detailed recommendations on the organisation and scope of the service. The most important of these were:

scheduled medical examinations should be available to each child at the age of six months, one year and two years;

in urban areas with a population of 5,000 or more, these scheduled medical examinations should be carried out in clinics by doctors on the medical officer's staff and, in some smaller towns, similar arrangements could operate;

the school should continue to be used as the basic centre for school health examinations, which would continue to be carried out by local medical officers;

in rural areas and in towns without clinics, the scheduled medical examinations for pre-school children should be undertaken by general practitioners under agreements with the health authorities;

the former aim of three routine medical examinations during a child's national school career should be replaced by a system under which there would be a comprehensive medical inspection of all children between the sixth and seventh birthdays, routine annual screening by the district nurse for vision, posture and cleanliness, audiometric testing of special groups, selected medical examinations of nine-year-old children and the examination in any year of a child referred by the parent, teacher or district nurse, or a child due for re-examination.

Section 66 of the Health Act, 1970 made the changes in the law necessary to give effect to recommendations of the working party. The programme provided initially for the development of the pre-school examination service in the towns with a population of 5,000 and over (to which it is generally confined still) and the restructuring of the school health examination service as recommended. The responsibility for giving effect to this programme is now, of course, one for the health boards.

In 1984, the number of examinations of infants at six months was 33,053 which was 67 per cent of those of that age. The number examined at twelve months was 11,612 and 5,599 were examined at two years. The 'take-up' at these ages was thus quite small. Of the children examined, about one-quarter were referred for further attention. This applied to each of the specified ages.

In the school health services, 121,101 children were examined in 1984, which was 21 per cent of national school children. Of these, 54,766 were new entrants to school. This was 74 per cent of the new entrants. Thirty-five per cent of the new entrants who were examined needed to be referred for further attention.[9]

Practically all new-born infants are screened by the laboratory at Temple Street Hospital, Dublin for rare metabolic disorders. The number screened in 1984 was 64,424. The ailments covered and the incidence of each found in that year were: phenylketonuria (one in 4,066), homocystinuria (one in 64,424), maple syrup urine disease (one in 32,212) galactosaemia (one in 12,885) and hypothyroidism (one in 4,602).[10]

HEALTH EDUCATION

The above measures relate to the actions of the public authorities in protecting the community against specific problems. However, over a much wider field, there is a responsibility on those authorities to aid and guide those in the community by protecting health and avoiding illness.[11] Much of this is, of course, done through the direct contacts between the medical officers, nurses and other staff of the health boards, and the people; much is also done through use of the mass media.

Because television, radio and the major newspapers are organised on a national basis, the major health publicity campaigns on these media were originally arranged direct by the Department of Health. New developments in the services were publicised and material issued from time to time on specific problems. The department also published a wide variety of leaflets.

As well as providing information and advice on particular diseases and health problems, the minister and the health boards have the responsibility to let the public have information on the health services available and on the rules governing eligibility for them. A general summary of the services is available from the department. Health boards have the responsibility to make information available on the local arrangements for the services.

The Health Education Bureau
The development of arrangements for health education was given a high priority in the health system. Recognition of this led in January 1975 to the establishment of the Health Education Bureau.[12] This was a corporate body with responsibility for organising health education programmes and for acting as the co-ordinating agency for the many voluntary bodies acting in this field. The bureau had a board of ten members, appointed by the Minister for Health, and employed its own staff to organise health education programmes. The bureau was dissolved at the end of 1987

and its work was taken over by a special unit in the Department of Health.

The Kilkenny Health Project

In 1984, the Irish Heart Foundation approached the Minister for Health for his agreement to a project aimed at studying and influencing the population of a defined area so as reduce in it the incidence of heart disease and related conditions. The county of Kilkenny was proposed. The minister agreed to this project and to its being co-financed by him (through the Medico-Social Research Board) and the foundation. The project commenced in October 1984 and is due to be completed in 1990.

The plan for the project provided for population surveys at its commencement and its conclusion and for a health promotion programme specifically related to the reduction of factors causing heart disease, which will continue for the duration of the project. The baseline survey was completed in August, 1986. Its purpose was to estimate the knowledge, attitudes and behaviour relevant to the development of coronary heart disease and to measure the levels of risk factors for that disease in a sample of the population of County Kilkenny. A total of 770 people was surveyed. A report on it, issued in November, 1986[13] stated 'in general the group surveyed displayed the social and demographic characteristics which would be expected of a random sample representative of the population of the county as a whole'. Among the points made in the report were:

over half of those surveyed had a family history of heart disease (either a parent or a sibling had had a heart attack),

almost 34 per cent of those surveyed were referred to their general practitioners because of high cholesterol levels (59 per cent in the case of women between fifty-five and sixty-five years),

81

24 per cent of males and 25 per cent of females between forty-five and fifty-four years of age and 42 per cent of males and 40 per cent of females between fifty-five and sixty-five years of age were referred because of high blood pressure (some of these were under treatment for the condition at the time, but most were not).

about one in five of those surveyed would be categorised as obese.

The project is continuing. Diets have been surveyed and the health promotion programme is going ahead, in collaboration with the South-Eastern Health Board, enthusiastically supported by many local interests. Clear objectives have been set. It is to be hoped that, when the second survey is carried out at the conclusion of the project, it will show results less startling than those above.

There is no reason to believe that those surveyed, or the people of Kilkenny as a whole, have, on average, health profiles any different from those for the rest of Ireland. Half of the country's deaths are due to heart disease and related conditions. It is to be hoped that the initiative started in Kilkenny will affect the community health protection programmes throughout the country in the furtherance of a general campaign to combat heart disease.

NOTES ON CHAPTER SIX

1. Health Statistics, 1986 (Department of Health), Table B5
2. Source: Department of Health
3. Ibid, Table B8
4. Under the National Drugs Advisory Board Establishment order, 1966 (S.I. 211), which was amended by a 1985 order (S.I. 220)
5. Source: National Co-ordinating Committee on Drug Abuse, First Annual Report, June 1986 (Pl 4285)
6. In pages 113 et seq., the report 'The Psychiatric Services – Planning for the Future' (1984) (Pl 3001) discusses this
7. The Tobacco Products (Control of Advertising, Sponsorship and Sales Promotion) (No. 2) Regulations, 1986 (S.I. 107)
8. The Child Health Services – Report of a Study Group, 1967 (Pr. 171)

9. Health Statistics, 1986, Tables B1 to B4
10. Ibid, Table B6
11. Under section 71 of the Health Act, 1970
12. Under the Health Education Bureau (Establishment) Order 1975 (S.I. 22)
13. Community Action towards Community Health: the Kilkenny Health Project, report published November 1986 by the project, Dean Street, Kilkenny.

CHAPTER SEVEN

Community health services programme

GENERAL MEDICAL AND NURSING SERVICES

General practitioner care

The responsibility of the health boards in organising care at general practitioner level extends only to those with full eligibility, representing 37 per cent of the population in September, 1987.

The genesis of the present general medical service is outlined in chapter four. The service in nearly all areas is based on agreements with participating doctors (rather than on the employment of doctors as officers, as in the case of the dispensary service). The form of agreement is a standard one. It sets out the obligations of the participating practitioner on the one hand and of the health board on the other. On the commencement of the new service, doctors in practice had an automatic right of entry. Other general practitioners did not have automatic right of entry. At present, doctors may acquire such a right after being in private practice in an area for five years. Otherwise, new doctors enter the scheme only where there is an accepted vacancy. Admission is on the basis of open competition. Group practice is allowed within the scheme and is encouraged by certain features of it.

Payment under the agreement is on the basis of fees for services, with the rates varying for surgery fees and for various kinds of domiciliary visits. There are higher rates for out-of-hours calls and for distant calls. The Minister for Health has recently initiated discussions with the Irish

Medical Organisation with a view to introducing a new system of payment based, at least partly, on capitation payments.

It is part of the normal contract that the medical practitioner will provide adequate surgery and waiting room facilities and that, in these arrangements, he will not discriminate between public and private patients. However, the use of premises such as clinics and dispensaries owned by the health board can be arranged. For islands and a few remote areas where choice of doctor is impracticable, the service is arranged through the employment of officers by the health boards.

A full description of the present arrangements is given in Appendix D.

Supply of drugs, medicines and appliances
Under the dispensary service, most of the doctors did their own dispensing from stocks of drugs which were kept at the dispensary and replenished by making official requisitions to the local authority. Where the doctor did not himself dispense, the drugs were issued by a pharmacist at the dispensary. This arrangement too was changed fundamentally in 1972. Retail pharmacists are the main channels of supply for drugs, medicines and appliances prescribed for eligible persons. Normally, a doctor participating in the service issues a prescription on a special form and this can be fulfilled by any pharmacist who has an agreement under the service (there are limitations on the list of the drugs which may be prescribed). The pharmacist is reimbursed for the cost of the drugs and is paid a fee for dispensing them. The prices and terms for supply to pharmacists of drugs by manufacturers and wholesalers are governed by an agreement made by the Department of Health with the Federation of Irish Chemical Industries.

Where the operation of this system of supply would cause hardship, either because there is no retail pharmaceutical chemist in an area or because of special circumstances in the case of a particular patient, it is part of the doctor's contract that he will arrange for the supply of drugs, etc. He is paid a special annual fee for this responsibility. He requisitions his drugs from a convenient retail pharmacist participating in the scheme.

These arrangements for the supply of drugs and medicines are also described in Appendix D.

General Medical Services (Payments) Board
The calculation of payments for the services of doctors and pharmacists under the service, the making of such payments, the verification of the accuracy and reasonableness of claims and the compilation of statistics and information on the services, are carried out for the health boards by a joint board, the General Medical Services (Payments) Board. Most of the members of this board are officers of health boards, the others being from the Department of Health.

The claims from doctors and pharmacists under the service are processed by computer and, on the basis of the information provided, the scheme is monitored regularly by the board. Each year it publishes a comprehensive report giving statistical information on the operation of the scheme. The following statistics are derived from the 1986 report.

Table 1: *Statistics on general medical service, 1986*

1. number of persons eligible for the service	1,323,035
2. percentage of estimated population	37.4
3. number of doctors in the service	1,512
4. number of these who are paid by fees......	1,481
5. number of persons covered per doctor	875
6. number of consultations (by doctors paid by fee)	
— surgery	7.0m
— domiciliary	1.5m
total...	8.5m
7. visiting rate (consultations divided by number eligible)......................................	6.4
8. number of pharmacies in the service........	1,105

9. number of prescription items dispensed in
   pharmacies 12.4m
10. number of dispensing doctors 354
11. number of patients for whom doctors
    dispense 145,582
12. total cost of fees to doctors £38.0m
13. cost per consultation £4.5
14. cost of consultations per person covered . £28.7
15. cost of supply of drugs and medicines
    — supplied by pharmacists on
      prescription £72.9m
    — supplied by dispensing doctors £6.6m
      total.. £79.5m
16. total cost of supply of drugs and medicines
    per person covered
    — supplied on prescription by
      pharmacists £62.1
    — supplied by dispensing doctors £45.3
17. total cost of service £117.5m
18. cost per eligible person £88.8

Drugs, medicines and appliances for persons without medical cards
The 'drug refund' scheme operated by the health boards[1] is
designed to insulate those with limited eligibility against
having to meet from their own resources heavy expenditure
on drugs, medicines and appliances which are prescribed by
doctors. Expenditure on drugs needed in any month over a
fixed limit (at present £28) is re-imbursed by the health
board. This refund scheme relates to drugs purchased through
the ordinary channels and is based on receipts obtained from
the retail pharmacists. The cost of the scheme in 1985 was
£6.6 million. The average number of claims per month was
17,362.

Drugs, etc. for long-term ailments
There are special arrangements for the supply of drugs,
medicines and appliances free of charge for persons suffering
from diseases or disabilities of a permanent or long-term
nature listed in regulations made by the minister.[2] This
scheme is available to all income groups. The list of diseases

and disabilities to which it applies are mental handicap, mental illness (in children under sixteen), phenylketonuria, cystic fibrosis, spina bifida, hydrocephalus, haemophilia, cerebral palsy, diabetes mellitus, diabetes insipidus, epilepsy, multiple sclerosis, muscular dystrophies, parkinsonism and acute leukaemia in children. This scheme also operates through the retail pharmacies, which supply the drugs prescribed and make claims for the cost of the drugs and their charges on the health boards. 43,177 persons availed themselves of this scheme in 1985 when it cost £8.2 million.

Home nursing
Nursing at community level was first developed by voluntary organisations, particularly the Queen's Institute of District Nursing in Ireland. Later there developed, side by side with the nurses of the voluntary agencies, a corps of public health nurses attached to the offices of the county medical officers of health, with duties mainly in the public health service. The Health Act, 1947,[3] gave health authorities power to appoint nurses for district duties and, in the nineteen-fifties, the authorities commenced the development of this service. Additional impetus was given by a circular issued by the department in June 1966.[4] The general objective of the service was stated as being to make public health nursing available to individuals and to families in each area throughout the country. More specifically:

> The object should be to provide such domiciliary midwifery services as may be necessary, general domiciliary nursing, particularly for the aged, and, at least equally important, to attend to the public health care of children, from infancy to the end of the school-going period. The nurses should provide health education in the home and assist local medical practitioners in the care of patients who need nursing care but who do not require treatment in an institution – whether for medical or social reasons. The aim should be to integrate the district nursing service with the general practitioner, hospital in-patient and out-

patient services, so that the nurse will be able to fulfil the important function of an essential member of the community health team, and carry out her duties in association with hospital staffs and other doctors in her district.

In the Health Act, 1970,[5] the objective of the home nursing service was defined as 'to give to (eligible) persons advice and assistance on matters relating to their health and to assist them if they are sick.

In 1985, there were 1,379 nurses in this service (including superintendents); that is one nurse for each 2,567 people. Each public health nurse is assigned to a district within the community care area and is responsible for preventive and curative health care within that area. In her work, the public health nurse can be involved in the community protection programme (child welfare clinics, etc.) and with the general practitioner service. The nurses are qualified in midwifery and have the formal duty to care for births at home but this is now of little significance. The cost of the service in 1985 was £20.1 million.

The Working Party on General Nursing reported in 1980 on this service.[6] It recommended an increase in the number of public health nurses and also the employment of other nurses to take over some of the work in home nursing.

MOTHERS, CHILDREN AND THE UNBORN

Maternity and infant care services
The health boards provide a service for medical attendance by general practitioners on maternity cases and on infants up to the age of six weeks for those with full eligibility and those in category 2 (as described in chapter five).[7] The service is provided through private medical practitioners under agreements with the health boards. This service also is based on the principle of choice of doctor. There is a standard form of agreement worked out by the department. The medical

practitioner undertakes to attend on any woman accepted by him. He attends during the ante-natal period, at the birth if he thinks it necessary (or if his services are called for by a midwife) and for the period of six weeks after the confinement. The services given normally include at least four visits before the confinement and two after it. Usually the same doctor will attend the infant, carrying out at least one medical examination during the first six weeks of life. The health board pays the fees for attendance on cases under the agreement.

In Dublin, an arrangement is made under which the staffs of the three maternity hospitals provide the same kind of services as are provided under the agreements with general practioners. The hospitals are, in such cases, viewed in the same way as individual participating private practitioners but when accepting services under such an arrangement the woman is not entitled to the services of any particular doctor on the hospital staff.

The number of cases using this service throughout the country in 1984 was 27,266, representing 42 per cent of the births in that year. However, less than one per cent of births took place at home. The service cost £1.8 million in 1985.

Family planning services
The Health (Family Planning) Act, 1979 made provision for family planning services and, with a view to ensuring that contraceptives are available only for the purpose, bona fide, of family planning or for adequate medical reasons, to regulate and control the sale, importation, manufacture and display of contraceptives. The act gave the Minister for Health a general duty to:

(a) secure the orderly organisation of family planning services, and
(b) provide a comprehensive natural family planning service, that is to say a comprehensive service for the provision of information, instruction, advice and consultation in relation to methods of family planning

that do not involve the use of contraceptives.

To this end, the act restricted family planning services, except for services exclusively for natural family planning, to health boards and other bodies approved by the minister.

In the original act, the sale of all contraceptives to the public was restricted to pharmacies and only on production of a prescription or authorisation signed by a doctor who was satisfied that they were for bona fide family planning purposes or for adequate medical reasons. The Health (Family Planning) (Amendment) Act, 1985 eased this restriction by allowing doctors (at their centres of practice), health boards (at health institutions), approved family planning clinics (at their premises) and hospitals providing maternity services or services for treating sexually transmitted diseases to sell contraceptives. It also removed, for contraceptive sheaths and spermicides supplied to persons over the age of eighteen years, the requirement that sales be restricted to doctors' authorisations or prescriptions.

The importation and sale of contraceptives was made subject to licence by the minister by the 1979 act and that act also allowed for regulations governing advertising and display.[8]

The health boards' programmes for family planning services did not develop very rapidly (in 1985 the total expenditure by the eight boards was £125,000) but, following the passage of the 1985 act, seven of the boards adopted plans for the development of family planning services. There are 17 family planning organisations (apart from the health boards) approved by the minister under section 2 of the 1979 act. Eight of these are in the greater Dublin area.

Abortion
The procuring of abortions and related activities (such as the administering of drugs or the use of instruments to procure abortion or the supplying of drugs or instruments to procure abortion) are prohibited under the Offences Against the Person Act, 1861. The Health (Family Planning) Act, 1979,

made it clear that nothing in it cut across this prohibition. In this respect, the following clause which was added to article 40.3 of the Constitution following a referendum in 1983, is relevant: 'The State acknowledges the right to life of the unborn and, with due regard to the equal right to life of the mother, guarantees in its laws to respect, and, as far as practicable, by its laws to defend and vindicate that right'.

DENTAL, OPHTHALMIC AND AURAL SERVICES

Dental services
The dental services arranged by the health boards[9] are concentrated on children (for defects noticed at child health examinations) and those with full eligibility. It has been the policy to restrict the services to these groups until, by adding to the personnel and generally improving the facilities, an adequate service is available for them. In the meantime, for persons insured under the Social Welfare Acts, dental (and optical and aural) benefits are available under a separate scheme administered by the Department of Social Welfare. The dental services of the health boards are provided mainly through whole-time dentists in their employment. The number of these increased from 210 in 1978 to 329 in 1984. In some areas, the services provided by this staff are supplemented by the part-time employment of private dental practitioners, who are usually paid on a sessional basis.

The work of the dental service is largely involved in combating the effects of existing dental decay but it is regarded as important that there should be as much concentration as possible on prevention. The instruction of children in good habits of dental care and oral hygiene is, therefore, a major aim of the service. Dental health campaigns, which are conducted by the Dental Health Education Committee of the Irish Dental Association, complement the activities of health boards in this field.

The following table[10] shows the numbers of treatments under this service in 1977 and 1984:

Table 2: *Services provided*	1977	1984
Children (mainly national school)		
number treated	276,982	310,781
fillings	259,399	251,680
extractions	205,965	176,242
orthodontic treatments	n.a.	5,005
Adults		
number treated	64,283	56,217
fillings	33,653	60,749
extractions	69,925	57,422
dentures	15,796	16,042

Expenditure on the service in 1985 came to £12.5 million.

Fluoridation

Fluoridation of public water supplies is the most important measure for preventing dental decay. Under the Health (Fluoridation of Water Supplies) Act, 1960, an obligation is placed on health boards to arrange for the fluoridation of piped public water supplies in their areas, the amount of fluorine added not to exceed one part per million. The local sanitary authorities operating the water supplies are obliged to co-operate as agents of the health boards in adding fluoride to the water. The scheme was commenced in the Dublin area in 1964 and has, at the time of writing, been extended to most of the piped water supply schemes in the country. Two-thirds of the population is now served by fluoridated water supplies (most of the remainder are in areas not served by piped supplies or in areas where the piped schemes are small and not suited to the installation of fluoridation equipment). Before fluoridation was introduced, detailed surveys were carried out on the incidence of dental caries in children. A national survey of children's dental health commissioned by the minister was carried out by University College, Cork in 1984.[11] The results, published in December 1986, showed that, while the general level of dental caries had declined among school children since the pre-fluoridation studies were carried out, the decline was greatest (and very significantly so) among children who were lifetime residents of fluoridated areas.

In some areas where there are not water supplies suitable for fluoridation, schemes have been brought in for applying fluoride by means of regular mouth-rinsing by the children, under suitable supervision.

Ophthalmic services
The health boards employ part-time ophthalmologists to examine eyes, to treat ailments and diseases and to prescribe spectacles. They may also arrange with medical practitioners and opticians in private practice for sight-testing of adults. Eligibility is the same as for the dental service. Spectacles are supplied by opticians under contract with the health boards. This service cost £3.8 million in 1985. Hospital in-patient and out-patient care for the eyes is part of the general hospital care programme described in chapter eleven.

The following table[12] shows the numbers of examinations and treatments under the ophthalmic service in 1977 and 1984:

Table 3: *Services provided*	*1977*	*1984*
Children (mainly national school)		
number examined	25,232	47,695
spectacles provided	27,392	19,011
Adults		
number examined	52,044	80,654
spectacles provided	55,155	76,266

Aural services
Consultant services for the treatment of ear defects are part of the general hospital care programme. The community health services programme is concerned specifically with the

assessment of hearing ability and the provision of hearing aids.[9] Specially trained public health nurses carry out audiometric tests and the health boards have arrangements with the National Rehabilitation Board to provide hearing aids for those eligible for the service.

The following statistics[13] relate to this service:

Table 4: *Services provided*	*1977*	*1984*
Children (pre-school and national school)		
number tested	179,415	164,385
number with significant defects	226	652
hearing aids supplied	650	193
Adults		
number examined by ENT		
specialists	n.a.	16,565
hearing aids supplied	1,568	1,677

The expenditure on this service in 1985 came to £0.8 million.

NOTES ON CHAPTER SEVEN

1. Under section 59(2) of the Health Act, 1970
2. Under section 59(3) of the Health Act, 1970
3. Section 102
4. Circular 27/66
5. Section 60
6. Report of Working Party on General Nursing, March 1980 (Prl 9156)
7. Under sections 62 and 63 of the Health Act, 1970
8. The Health (Family Planning) Regulations, 1986 (S.I. No. 248 of 1986) deal with these and some other matters
9. Under section 67 of the Health Act, 1970
10. Sources: Health Statistics, 1980, Table C6; Health Statistics, 1986, Table C6
11. Children's Dental Health in Ireland, 1984 – A survey conducted on behalf of the Minister for Health by University College, Cork (Pl 4530)

12. Sources: Health Statistics, 1980, Table C8; Health Statistics, 1986, Table C8
13. Sources: Health Statistics, 1980, Table C9; Health Statistics, 1986, Table C9

CHAPTER EIGHT

Community welfare programme

Welfare services are the responsibility of a number of government departments and of several subordinate authorities. However, because many aspects of welfare are closely linked with health care – particularly in relation to children and the aged – the health agencies have developed, and are continuing to develop, an increasing role in the provision of personal welfare services which come within the general scope of the health agencies. Specifically in the case of income maintenance services, those dealt with by the Department of Social Welfare are not covered.

CASH BENEFITS

Disabled persons allowances and mobility allowances
Maintenance allowances are paid by health boards to disabled persons over sixteen years of age who are unable to provide for their own maintenance.[1] The maximum rate for these allowances is fixed in regulations made by the Minister for Health. These allowances are paid only to persons whose disability has lasted, or is expected to last, for one year from its onset. Those maintained in institutions are not eligible for the allowances. There were 24,019 beneficiaries under this scheme on 31 December 1984.[2]

For severely handicapped persons aged between sixteen and sixty-six years of age who are unable to walk and who would benefit from occasional trips away from home, there is a scheme for the payment of mobility allowances, subject to a means test.

The cost of these allowances for disabled and handicapped people in 1985 was £53.4 million.

97

Infectious diseases allowances
Health boards also pay maintenance allowances to persons receiving treatment for infectious diseases.[3] Primarily, this scheme is applicable to those with tuberculosis, but it also covers some other diseases (see page 212). The scheme is applicable to persons undergoing treatment (to the satisfaction of the local medical officer) who are unable to make 'reasonable and proper provision for their own maintenance or the maintenance of their dependants'. The scales of allowances are fixed by the minister and are varied from time to time in line with changes in allowances under social welfare schemes.

Allowances may also be paid to carriers of the diseases concerned. If, through taking precautions against the spread of infection, a person is rendered incapable of carrying on his or her ordinary occupation and is thereby 'unable to make reasonable and proper provision for his (or her) own maintenance or the maintenance of his (or her) dependants', an allowance may be paid. A case in point would be a typhoid carrier employed in a restaurant who is directed to give up the handling of food.

The cost of infectious diseases allowances in 1985 was £0.5 million. There were 181 recipients of them in 1984.

Maternity cash grants
Cash grants in respect of confinements are paid by health boards for women with full eligibility.[4] The rate of the grant is £8 for each child. These grants are distinct from (and may be supplementary to) the maternity benefits given for insured persons under the Social Welfare Acts. They cost £80,000 in 1985. The number of grants paid in 1984 was 6,108.

Blind welfare allowances
Health boards pay allowances additional to the blind pensions payable by the Department of Social Welfare and to the disabled persons allowances referred to above in the case of necessitous blind persons. Such allowances were paid to 1,087

blind persons in 1984. Expenditure on them came to £1 million in 1985.

Constant care allowances
There is a scheme for the payment of 'constant care' allowances to the parents of disabled children maintained at home. It is paid irrespective of the means of the parents. Allowances were being paid for 6,365 children under this scheme on 31 December 1984. The cost in 1985 was £5.1 million.

Supplementary welfare allowances
The home assistance service which was the responsibility of local authorities and was under the general control of the Department of Social Welfare was replaced on 1 July 1977 by a new scheme of supplementary welfare allowances. This scheme is operated by the health boards but is governed by regulations made by the Minister for Social Welfare.

WELFARE SERVICES

Home helps
The home assistance service had traditionally been used in an ancillary way to the health services in the maintenance at home of the aged and of sick or infirm persons. More specific authority for this purpose was given to the health boards under the Health Act, 1970[5]. The boards were given a broad power to make arrangements for the maintenance at home of sick or infirm persons and certain other categories – with specific reference to cases which would otherwise need to be maintained in an institution. The health boards also have the power to give grants to voluntary agencies providing services 'similar or ancillary to' the services of the boards.[6] Under these provisions, health boards themselves employ home helps and make grants to voluntary agencies. They also make grants to voluntary agencies towards the cost of meals-on-wheels. For tuberculosis patients living at home,

food, clothing, medicines and appliances may be provided under a special scheme. There are also arrangements for supplying milk for expectant and nursing mothers and children under five years of age in the 'full eligibility' category.[7]

Table 1 shows the numbers benefiting from these services[8] at 31 December 1984

Table 1: *Welfare services—numbers benefiting*

home helps.. 10,790
'meals-on-wheels'.................................. 18,212
domiciliary TB scheme.......................... 954
milk for mothers and children............. 21,401

The cost of the services in 1985 was £17.9 million.

CHILD CARE

Alongside the services for the care of children's health referred to in other chapters, the Department of Health and the health boards have been given an increased role in the care of disadvantaged children. This arose partly from the transfer in 1982 from the Minister for Justice to the Minister for Health of functions under the Adoption Acts, 1952 to 1976, and the transfer to him in 1983 from the Minister for Education of non-educational functions relating to industrial schools (except for those at Finglas West in Dublin and Clonmel). However, the traditional roles of the department and that of the health boards—taken over from the local authorities—relating to fostered children have also expanded.

Foster care and residential care
Orphans and children who are deserted by their parents and who have no one else to look after them may be placed in foster care (boarded out) by health boards.[9] A child whose parents cannot provide the necessities of life may also be boarded-out, with the agreement of the parents. The fostering

arrangement normally lasts until sixteen years of age, but the health board may, after this age, continue it for the completion of a child's education. The regulations require that contract be entered into between the board and the foster-parent and specify conditions as respects the suitability of the latter and certain facilities which must be available. Officers of the health board (generally social workers or public health nurses) and Department of Health inspectors may visit boarded-out children and the foster-homes.

While fostering is the preferred arrangement, health boards may also pay for the keep of children in 'approved schools'. These are industrial schools and orphanages, generally maintained by religious orders. A health board may also arrange for the placing of a fostered child in 'any suitable trade calling or business'.

On 31 December 1983, there were 2,534 children in care. Of these 1,267 were fostered out by the health boards, and 1,186 were placed by the boards in residential accommodation. Seventy-one were in private fosterage and ten were under supervision at home. During that year, there were in all 3,595 admissions into care. Table 2 below shows the primary reasons for admission.[10]

Table 2: *Admission into care*   %

one parent family unable to cope	1,133	31
neglect of child	597	17
short-term crisis	490	14
abuse of child (physical, emotional or sexual)	325	9
marital disharmony	322	9
child awaiting adoption	256	7
child abandoned	248	7
child out of control	172	5
both parents dead	52	1

The cost of the fostering service in 1985 was £2.5 million and the payments for children in residential homes came to

£6.3 million. In additional grants paid by the health boards to 283 pre-school day care centres (attended by 6,681 children) cost £0.5 million.

Protection of children

The Children Acts, 1908 to 1957, are a comprehensive code for the protection of children against various forms of victimisation. Health boards are directly concerned only with the sections of the acts which relate to the supervision of children placed in foster-homes, or placed in employment in certain circumstances.[11] The intention to receive a child under sixteen as a foster-child for reward (or if the child is illegitimate, without reward) must be notified to the health board and the board has the responsibility to satisfy itself about the suitability of the home. It must arrange for the regular visiting of the child in the home.

Where any body or person, except a parent or other relative, proposes to send a child under eighteen years of age away for employment, the health board must also be notified and it has similar powers of supervision and visiting as respects that child. Health boards may contribute to the funds of any society for the prevention of cruelty to children.[12]

Children (Care and Protection) Bill, 1985

This bill, which was introduced by the Minister for Health, was designed to update and extend the law relating to the care and protection of children, particularly those who are neglected or otherwise at risk. The second stage of this bill was passed in the Dail on 23 January 1986 but it had not proceeded further before the dissolution of the twenty-fourth Dail in January 1987. Complications on some of the bill's provisions had arisen from a judgement in the Supreme Court in 1985. The present government has indicated its intention of introducing a similar bill.

Adoption

The legal adoption of children is provided for in the Adoption Act, 1952. That act established a body, An Bord Uchtala (the Adoption Board), with the function of approving of and registering adoptions. The board does not itself arrange adoptions but registers societies with this as their object. Before registering an adoption, the board satisfies itself as to the suitability of the adopters and may refuse an adoption order if it thinks fit. The effect of an adoption order is that a child acquires the surname of the adopters and, generally speaking, is placed in the same position as if he or she had been born to them legitimately. Where a child fostered under the provisions described above is adopted by the foster-parents, the health board is no longer liable for its maintenance but, so that there would be no disincentive on the part of the foster-parents to adopt a child if they so wished, the health board is authorised to continue to contribute to the maintenance of the child as if still fostered out.[13]

From the commencement of the 1952 act on 1 January 1953, to 31 December 1986 a total of 34,617 adoption orders were made by the board. The numbers of adoptions have dropped in recent years – from 1,195 in 1984 to 885 in 1985 and 800 in 1986. Most adoptions (64 per cent in 1986) arise from placements by adoption societies. Family adoptions – generally the natural mother and her husband – account for most of the rest (27 per cent in 1986) with small numbers placed by health boards and by the natural mother.[14]

A committee set up by the Minister for Health to review the adoption services reported in 1984.[15] It recommended many changes in the laws and procedures. Amendments arising from these are proposed in a bill currently before the Oireachtas.

Expenditure on adoption services in 1985 came to £0.5 million.

CARE OF THE AGED

The care of the aged is not a monopoly of any one part of the health services. Those old people who are living at home

103

have available to them the range of services referred to elsewhere, subject to the general rules about eligibility. They similarly have access to the acute general hospital services. Many aged people, however, reach the stage when they can no longer be looked after in a private dwelling and must be taken into a home. For such of these as are unable to arrange this from their own resources, the health boards provide maintenance.

As described in earlier chapters, the institutional care of the aged was traditionally provided in the county homes which were adapted from some of the nineteenth-century workhouses. An inter-departmental committee on the care of the aged, which reported in 1968,[16] recommended that the concept of these homes should be abandoned and that a system should be developed under which the need of the aged for institutional care would be carefully assessed, steps would be taken to assign patients to the most appropriate form of care and every effort would be made to rehabilitate patients and restore them to the community. The committee recommended that provision for the aged should be made in four main types of accommodation – general hospitals, geriatric assessment units, long-stay hospital units and welfare homes. These recommendations form the basis of current policy on the services.

On 31 December 1984, some 14,098 persons were in care in geriatric units and homes, divided as shown in Table 3.

Table 3: *Persons in care*

Health board geriatric hospitals and homes	7,038
Health board welfare homes	1,458
Voluntary approved nursing homes	2,972
Other private nursing homes......................	2,630

The average occupation rate in the hospitals and homes was 94 per cent. About 70 per cent of the patients were over 75 years of age. While most had some illness, about a quarter were classified as being in care for social reasons. 65 per cent of the patients were female.[17]

Expenditure on care in welfare homes for the aged came to £7.4 million in 1985. (This does not include the cost of care in health board geriatric hospitals, units and homes. This is included in the figure for the general hospital programme).

NOTES ON CHAPTER EIGHT

1. Under section 69 of the Health Act, 1970
2. The source for this statistic and those relating to the other allowances is Health Statistics, 1986, Table D1
3. Under section 44 of the Health Act, 1947
4. Under section 64 of the Health Act, 1970
5. Section 61
6. Under section 65 of the Health Act, 1953
7. Under section 65 of the Health Act, 1970
8. Source: Health Statistics, 1986, Table D3
9. Under sections 55 and 56 of the Health Act, 1953
10. The source of these statistics is *Children in Care, 1983,* published by the Department of Health.
11. Part I of the Children Act, 1908, as amended (mainly by section 57 of the Health Act, 1953 and sections 2 and 3 of the Children Act, 1957)
12. Under section 65(2) of the Health Act, 1953
13. Under section 55(9) of the Health Act, 1953
14. Source: annual reports of the Adoption Board
15. Adoption: Report of the Review Committee on the Adoption Services, May 1984 (Pl 2467)
16. The Care of the Aged – Report of the Interdepartmental Committee, 1968 (Prl 777).
17 The source of these statistics is Health Statistics, 1986, Tables G15– G18

CHAPTER NINE

Psychiatric programme

Earlier chapters described the separate origins of the services for the mentally ill and the convergence of these services and the general health services into the same administrative structure. This is now complete, with the health boards responsible for the mental health service. In its nature too, the mental health service has tended towards becoming more like the general health services, although the facilities for the psychiatric service are still mainly based on the nineteenth-century hospitals within which it developed.

The estimated non-capital expenditure on the psychiatric programme in 1985 was £147 million. Capital expenditure came to £6.3 million.

ELIGIBILITY FOR MENTAL HOSPITAL SERVICES

The rules on eligibility for care in and at psychiatric hospitals are on the whole the same as for general hospitals. For children under sixteen years of age, the full range of services is, however, available irrespective of their own or their parents' means. Health boards make payments, as in the case of general hospital care, for persons going to private psychiatric hospitals or homes for in-patient treatment.

Reception and maintenance of patients
The Mental Treatment Act, 1945 is currently the basic statute on the mental health service. The 1945 act specifies three categories of patients in psychiatric hospitals, voluntary patients, temporary patients and those certified as 'persons of unsound mind'.[1] Most patients in psychiatric hospitals are

106

now admitted voluntarily and very few under the procedure for persons of unsound mind. Details of the mode of admission for each class are specified in the act, which also deals with the procedures and restrictions in relation to the detention of patients and the patients' rights of appeal in relation to detention. A short summary of these provisions is given in Appendix E.

The Commission of Inquiry on Mental Illness

The Commission of Inquiry on Mental Illness was appointed by the Minister for Health in 1961 to examine and report on the health services available for the mentally ill and on changes thought necessary or desirable in legislation. It reported in 1966, making wide-ranging recommendations.[2]

The Commission:

emphasised the need for active and early treatment of mental illness and for the integration of psychiatry and general medicine, and thus favoured a concept of psychiatric units in, or associated with, general hospitals;

for long-stay patients, recommended that mental hospitals should be regarded not merely as centres for custodial care, but that planned and purposeful activity for the patients should be featured, with a view to their rehabilitation and restoration to the community as far as possible;

thought that the aim should be to have the number of long-stay places halved in fifteen years;

recommended that private psychiatric hospitals should, like the voluntary general hospitals, be involved in providing services for the health authorities;

stressed the need to give priority to the development of out-patient services;

107

thought that general practitioners should be encouraged to take a greater interest and a more active role in psychiatry and that public health personnel should play a greater part than heretofore in the promotion of mental health;

made specific recommendations on the problems of children, adolescents and the aged and on alcoholism, drug addiction, epilepsy and other special classes such as homicidal patients, psychopaths and sexual deviates;

advocated improved measures for prevention and research and for the education and training of professional staff and others in relation to psychiatry; emphasised the need for more time being given to the study of psychiatry in the curricula of the medical schools;

recommended a number of amendments in the legislation dealing with the mentally ill, mainly designed towards making the reception and detention of most psychiatric patients more informal;

recommended more flexible provisions in relation to the boarding-out of patients.

The recommendations of the commission have largely been followed in the development of policy on the psychiatric services. Its recommendations were implemented, for example, in the transfer of the responsibility for the Central Mental Hospital, Dundrum to the Eastern Health Board and in the co-ordination with the private psychiatric hospitals, particularly in the Dublin area.

Planning for the Future
A new review of the psychiatric services was conducted by a study group of officers of the Department of Health, the health boards and the Medico-Social Research Board which

was set up by the minister in 1981. Its report *Planning for the Future,* was published in 1984.[3] It surveyed the incidence of mental illness and the arrangements for treating it and made recommendations for future planning.

The group's report stated:

> The main thrust of our conclusions is that the psychiatric needs of the community should be met by a comprehensive and integrated service made up of a number of treatment components and largely located in the community. A number of changes are necessary if this objective is to be achieved. In particular, there must be a decided shift in the pattern of care from an institutional setting with close links between psychiatric and other community services.[4]

The group commented that its conclusions were very much in the spirit of the recommendations of the 1961 commission. The minister, Barry Desmond, announced on the publication of the report that it was the government's intention to implement the recommendations contained in it.[5]

In-patient care
The health board hospitals provide the basis for over 80 per cent of in-patient care for the mentally ill. There were twenty-two health board psychiatric hospitals in 1984 (two have since been closed). On 31 December in that year, there were 10,880 patients in these hospitals. Fifteen special units provided by the health boards in their general hospitals and in other institutions had 560 patients and 12 private psychiatric hospitals accommodated 948 patients. The Central Mental Hospital, Dundrum had 96 patients – making a total in hospital on that date of 12,484.[6] There has been a continuing decline in the numbers in these hospitals. In 1963, the total was 19,810 and in 1971 it was 16,661.[7] The reports of the Medico-Social Research Board on its studies on the activities of psychiatric hospitals and units give very detailed information on admissions. For 1984, the study[8] showed that the admission rate was 8.4 per 1,000 population. Three-

quarters of the admissions were due to the following three categories of psychiatric illness:

depressive disorders (2.3 per 1,000 population)

alcohol abuse and alcoholic psychosis (2.1 per 1,000).

schizophrenia (1.8 per 1,000).

Community care

Out-patient clinics are arranged in the health board hospitals. In the year to 31 May 1984, the number of patients who attended these was 30,886. Facilities for day care were available in 32 hospitals and other centres and were attended by 963 patients. Hostels for the mentally ill were provided by the health boards in 99 centres. These accommodated 791. Community workshops were provided in 39 centres and were attended by 1,170 persons.[9] Comparable statistics are not available on out-patient care at the private psychiatric hospitals, nor on the care of mentally ill patients by general practitioners.

These numbers of patients cared for in the community, if totalled, give a figure much higher than that for in-patients. However, there is overlapping among the above figures for out-patient care and there can be overlapping between them and the figure for in-patients. Nevertheless, they are a good indicator of the extent to which community care has replaced institutional care for the mentally ill.

NOTES ON CHAPTER NINE

1. The Health (Mental Services) Act, 1981 is designed to replace much of the 1945 act. It has not been brought into force and it is being reviewed (Planning for the Future, par 1.8, page 3)
2. Report of Commission of Inquiry on Mental Illness, 1965 (Pr 9181)
3. The Psychiatric Services – Planning for the Future: Report of a Study Group on the Psychiatric Services, 1984 (Pl 3001)
4. Introduction to the report, par. 6, page viii.
5. Foreword to the report, page (iii)
6. Source: Health Statistics, 1986 Tables E1 to E3.

7. Planning for the Future, table 7 page 164
8. Activities of Irish Psychiatric Hospitals and Units, 1984; Medico-Social Research Board
9. Health Statistics, 1986, Tables E7 to E14.

CHAPTER TEN

Programme for the handicapped

MENTAL HANDICAP

We have seen in earlier chapters how responsibility for the care of the mentally handicapped was successively shunted from houses of industry to lunatic asylums, to workhouses and to county homes and how a policy for caring for the mentally handicapped in special homes and other institutions evolved in the nineteen-fifties and nineteen-sixties. This policy is described in the Report of the Commission of Enquiry on Mental Handicap which was published in 1965.[1] The care of the mentally handicapped is now based mainly on specialist residential centres, mostly operated by voluntary bodies and on a variety of community services operated by health boards and other agencies. The proportion of the mentally handicapped kept in mental hospitals is now relatively small, as Figure 1 (based on 1985 figures) shows:

Figure 1: *Care of mentally handicapped*

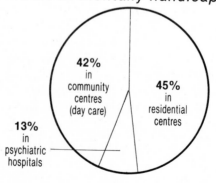

Residential centres and other units[2]

There are 60 residential centres, 49 under the control of voluntary bodies (financed mainly by state funds) and 11 operated by health boards. The centres range in size from some with over 300 places down to small units catering for less than ten. Religious orders and lay voluntary bodies have been involved in the development of the centres and in their administration.

A total of 9,834 persons were cared for by the homes and other units for the mentally handicapped in 1985 (this figure does not include about 1,500 mentally handicapped persons in psychiatric hospitals). The total is sub-divided in Table 1.

Table 1: *Care of mentally handicapped*

Setting	Under 15 years	Over 15 years	All Ages
Maintained in homes	961	4138	5099
Hostels and lodgings	98	675	773
Day attenders	956	3006	3962
Totals	2015	7819	9834

Of those in care, 20 per cent were classified as having mild handicap, the remainder being moderate, severe or profound.

Eligibility for services

The normal rules for entitlement to hospital services nominally apply in relation to eligibility for the care of the mentally handicapped, but the care of all children up to the age of sixteen is free without reference to the parents' means. As those over sixteen would have their income assessed in their own right, without reference to that of the parents or other relatives, it will be clear that very few mentally handicapped persons are in category 3 as defined on page 66 and thus outside the scope of entitlement to the full range of the services.

113

Census of the mentally handicapped

The Medico-Social Research Board carried out a census of mentally handicapped persons in Ireland in 1981. A total of 22,979 were enumerated in this census as having some degree of mental handicap, representing a prevalence rate of 6.7 per 1,000 total population. However, four in ten of this total (9,443) were identified as borderline or as having mild mental handicap, most of these being in the community rather than in residential care.[3]

Expenditure

Public expenditure on the care of the mentally handicapped came to £104.8 million in 1985.

OTHER HANDICAPS

A wide range of physical and psychological handicaps comes within the scope of the programme for the handicapped. These include congenital conditions and conditions caused by accidents and the after-effects of disease. The health boards operate programmes for the assessment and care of the blind, the deaf and persons otherwise handicapped. The cost of these in 1985 was £15 million. Many voluntary bodies are involved in caring for special groups of the handicapped in different ways.[4]

In the current year (1988), health boards are to develop services to aid in the mobility of the seriously disabled. This will replace arrangements operated through the Revenue Commissioners for tax concessions for cars for the disabled.

REHABILITATION

Health boards are required to make available a service for the training of disabled persons (whether mentally or physically handicapped) for employment and for making arrangements with employers for placing disabled persons in suitable employment.[5] A number of other bodies are active in this field. The National Rehabilitation Board is a body set up by the minister under the Health (Corporate Bodies) Act, 1961 to advise him, to co-ordinate the work of other bodies engaged in rehabilitation and to initiate schemes for rehabilitation. The board provides vocational assessment and guidance services, arranges vocational training and provides a job placement service. It is associated with the Sisters of Mercy in the operation of the National Medical Rehabilitation Centre, Dun Laoghaire.

Services are provided in several centres throughout the country by voluntary organisations and health boards, the most prominent being the Rehabilitation Institute, Dublin. In 1984, there were 63 centres (25 of which were operated by the institute) with places for 3,706.[6]

Grants from the EC Social Fund for the training of the handicapped have been available since 1974. They totalled £18 million in 1984.[7]

NOTES ON CHAPTER TEN

1. Report of Commission of Inquiry on Mental Handicap, 1965 (Pr 8234)
2. The basis of the succeeding paragraphs is Tables F3 and F4, Health Statistics, 1986
3. Census of Mental Handicap in the Republic of Ireland, 1981, Medico-Social Research Board, page 17
4. On page 296 et seq of the *Administration Year Book and Diary, 1988*, published by the Institute of Public Administration, such bodies are listed
5. Section 68 of Health Act, 1970
6. Source: table F5, Health Statistics, 1986, which lists the centres
7. Page 51, Health Statistics, 1986

CHAPTER ELEVEN

General hospital care programme

The general hospital care programme is concerned broadly with that part of the health services in which care is provided for acute cases in or at hospitals. The programme includes care at specialised hospitals, such as the maternity hospitals and the fever hospitals, but does not cover care for acute conditions at psychiatric hospitals (some general hospitals, however, have psychiatric units).

The programme is the most expensive branch of the health services, absorbing 51 per cent of the non-capital expenditure in 1985 (when expenditure on it totalled £637 million) and 75 per cent of the capital expenditure.

The public hospital system is made up of two groups, the health board hospitals and the public voluntary hospitals. In 1984, there were 95 health board hospitals, with a total bed complement of 9,548 and 41 voluntary hospitals, with a total bed complement of 7,787. In addition, there were 16 private hospitals with a total of 1,522 beds. In all, 608,270 patients were discharged from these hospitals in that year, 93% from the public hospitals and 7% from the private hospitals. The public hospitals also catered for 1,574,489 attendances at 70,779 out-patient sessions.[1]

THE HEALTH BOARD HOSPITALS

These hospitals are administered by the health boards and are financed from their budgets. The group is made up of regional hospitals, county hospitals, district hospitals, fever hospitals and orthopaedic hospitals.

116

The regional hospitals

These are hospitals with specialised units not found in most county hospitals. In 1984 there were ten hospitals classified as regional, most of them being teaching hospitals, they included the major general hospitals in Cork, Galway, Limerick, Sligo and Waterford and maternity hospitals in Cork and Limerick. There were 3,021 beds in, and 119,616 patients were discharged from, the regional hospitals in 1984. The average duration of stay was 7.5 days and the bed occupancy ratio was 82 per cent.[2]

To fulfil their special role, these hospitals are well staffed with consultants (including some in specialised categories), other medical staff, nurses and other professionals.

The county hospitals

The origins of the county hospitals are referred to in earlier chapters. Since 1970, the capacity and number of these hospitals have changed but little (in 1981, the Sligo hospital was classified as regional, reducing the number of county hospitals). The average county hospital has about 140 beds and provides general medical and surgical care and maternity services.

Since 1970, there has been a considerable increase in the numbers treated in the county hospitals, as shown in Table 1.

Table 1: *Numbers treated in county hospitals*[3]

	1970	1984
Number of hospitals	24	23
Beds	3,117	3,189
Patients discharged	91,142	135,009
Average duration of stay	10.4 days	6.6 days
Patient throughput per bed	29.2	42.3
Percentage occupancy	83.4	76.9

Originally, the staffing of the county hospitals at consultant level was based on one physician and one surgeon but, as their role has developed, the hospitals generally have more than one in each of these categories and additional consultants for specialised purposes.

The district hospitals

These are small hospitals with facilities for medical care and minor surgery and in some cases for obstetrics. They are staffed by general practitioners. In 1984, there were 53 district hospitals averaging 46 beds. Some have been closed since.

In contrast to the county hospitals, the number of patients cared for in the district hospitals has dropped substantially – from 27,252 in 1970 to 19,635 in 1984. In that period, the number of beds in the hospitals increased from 1,998 to 2,445 but the average duration of stay rose from 20 days to 37 days.[4] This reflects a change whereby most of these hospitals have become long-stay institutions for chronic conditions.

Other health board hospitals

There are four fever hospitals. Cherry Orchard Hospital, County Dublin is the major hospital, with 282 beds. The other three – at Cork, Galway and Killarney – had a total of 132 beds in 1984. 5,893 patients were discharged from these hospitals in that year, the occupancy of beds being 46.7 per cent.[5]

There are orthopaedic hospitals in Croom, Co. Limerick, Navan, Co. Meath, Kilcreene, Co. Kilkenny and Gurrena-braher, Cork. In 1984, these had 477 beds. 9,719 patients were discharged in that year compared with 5,365 in 1970. The average duration of stay dropped over the same period from 37 days to 13 days. The occupancy of beds in 1984 was 71 per cent.

The law on health board hospitals

The law governing the provision and maintenance of hospitals by the health boards is contained in Part III of the Health Act, 1970, which gives a general authority for the provision and maintenance of hospitals and specifies the conditions

118

under which changes can be made or institutions discontinued. The employment of staff for these hospitals is governed by the general provisions on officers and servants in health boards referred to in chapter fourteen.

THE PUBLIC VOLUNTARY HOSPITALS

The following extract from the report of the Consultative Council on the General Hospital Services (the Fitzgerald Report)[6] describes the development of the voluntary hospital system:

1.2 The Irish voluntary hospital movement had its origins in the early decades of the 18th century and, because of the penal restrictions of the period on religious communities, was initially entirely lay in character. Philanthropic individuals, moved by the conditions of the sick poor, voluntarily took on themselves the task of establishing and running hospitals and raising money for them. It was a form of charity to the public not available in Ireland since the closure of the monasteries following the Reformation. On the other hand, in Britain, under Elizabethan legislation, a system of rate-supported public parochial assistance, including provision for the poor infirm, had been devised, but it had not been extended to Ireland.

1.3 The development of the Irish voluntary hospital was almost entirely confined to the city areas, particularly to Dublin. The movement depended largely for its support on the commercial and professional classes, an element not significantly represented in rural areas. Many of the hospitals had a short career, because of lack of continued financial support, but some of the earliest voluntary hospitals have survived to the present day. In Dublin, the Charitable Infirmary, Jervis Street; Dr Steevens' Hospital;

119

Mercer's Hospital; the Rotunda Maternity Hospital; the Royal Hospital for Incurables and the Meath Hospital all have early 18th century origins, and some of them were the earliest hospitals of their type in the world. The Dublin House of Industry, which eventually included in its complex of buildings the Richmond, Whitworth and Hardwicke Hospitals, started developing in 1773 and now forms St Laurence's Hospital. The North Infirmary and the South Infirmary, Cork also date from the same period as do, among others, the County and City Infirmary, Waterford.

1.4 During the first half of the 19th century the voluntary hospital movement was still the main force in providing for the sick poor. In Dublin, Sir Patrick Dun's Hospital, the Coombe Maternity Hospital, the Adelaide Hospital, the Royal City of Dublin Hospital, the Royal Victoria Eye and Ear Hospital and the National Children's Hospital, Harcourt Street, came into existence. Barrington's Hospital was opened in Limerick. A significant influence on voluntary hospital development was the growth of more liberal political attitudes and the lifting of restrictions on the Catholic community, thus allowing the foundation of a number of new Irish Orders of Religious dedicated to the care of the sick poor. The Irish Sisters of Charity founded St Vincent's Hospital, Dublin, in 1834. The Sisters of Mercy opened the Mercy Hospital in Cork in 1857 and the Mater Misericordiae Hospital in Dublin in 1861. A great expansion of these and other Orders took place from then on, resulting in a most important contribution to the Irish hospital provision, among other examples of the charitable actions of these Orders.'

Many of the voluntary hospitals mentioned are there still. They have been joined by a new group – those hospitals which are administered by boards established by the Minister for Health under the Health (Corporate Bodies) Act, 1961. These are: Beaumont Hospital, St James's Hospital and St Luke's Hospital, all in Dublin (another will be added when a new hospital planned for Tallaght, Co. Dublin is built). Perhaps these are not voluntary in the sense of the original group of hospitals but they are sufficiently close to them in their nature to justify 'voluntary' as a generic description for non-health board public hospitals. For the whole group of voluntary general hospitals, there was, between 1979 and 1984 an increase in the number of discharges of patients from 167,574 to 182,334 and a decrease in the average duration of stay from 10.1 days to 8.7 days. The bed occupancy ratio in 1984 was 81 per cent.[7]

The voluntary public hospitals may be divided into four categories – general teaching hospitals, general non-teaching hospitals, cottage hospitals and special hospitals.

General teaching hospitals
These are the major voluntary hospitals in Dublin and Cork. In 1984, there were 11 in Dublin, with a total of 3,504 beds. These, separately and in combinations, provided the teaching facilities for the three medical schools in the city. Four voluntary hospitals in Cork, with 598 beds, provided similar facilities for the medical school there, complementing the health board's regional hospital.[8]

General non-teaching and cottage hospitals
Seven of the voluntary hospitals, with a total of 1,034 beds in 1984 were in this category. They ranged in size from 33 beds in Monkstown Hospital, Co. Dublin (which has since been closed) to 360 in Our Lady of Lourdes Hospital, Drogheda. They differ in the ranges of care provided. The cottage hospitals, of which there are two, are quite small and provide a limited service.[9]

Special hospitals
In 1984, there were 16 specialised public voluntary hospitals – four maternity hospitals, three children's hospitals, three

cancer hospitals, two eye, ear and throat hospitals, and four orthopaedic hospitals. The three Dublin maternity hospitals – the Coombe, the Rotunda and the National Maternity – catered for 19,696 births in 1984, about 31 per cent of the total for the country. The children's hospitals are in Dublin, the largest being Our Lady's, Crumlin. The three hospitals catered for 27,381 patients in 1984. The three cancer hospitals are also in Dublin, as are the orthopaedic hospitals including, the National Rehabilitation Centre.[10]

JOINT SERVICES

Blood transfusion
A nation-wide blood transfusion service, including the processing and supply of blood derivatives and blood products, is provided for the various hospitals by the Blood Transfusion Service Board. This is a board of twelve members appointed by the minister. Donation of blood is organised by the board on a voluntary basis and the board's running expenses are met by contributions from the hospitals for the blood supplied.[11]

Sterile requisites
The Hospitals Joint Services Board, also set up under the Health (Corporate Bodies) Act, 1961 provides a service for the supply of sterile requisites to hospitals and has also established a laundry to provide a centralised service for Dublin hospitals. The board has fifteen members who are appointed by the minister.[12]

Ambulance services
The health boards operate ambulance services. The boards have a general power to provide ambulances or other means of transport for the conveyance of patients.[13] In some areas, the fire brigades operate the ambulance service as agents of the health boards. Where necessary, army helicopters are used, on a repayment basis, to convey patients.

TOWARDS RATIONALISING THE HOSPITAL SYSTEM

Reference is made on page 22 to the First Report of the Hospitals Commission which proposed a reduction of the number of hospitals and their better organisation. This recommendation was shelved but since 1960 there has been movement towards restructuring the hospital system. The first initiative came from seven of the Dublin voluntary hospitals – the Adelaide, Dr Steevens, the Meath, Mercer's, the National Children's, Harcourt Street, the Royal City of Dublin and Sir Patrick Dun's – which sought federation with a view to their ultimate amalgamation in a new hospital. They asked the minister, Sean MacEntee, to sponsor legislation to facilitate this. He agreed and the Hospitals Federation and Amalgamation Act, 1961, was enacted. These hospitals were joined under a statutory council. However, little movement had been made towards actual amalgamation when broader initiatives towards re-organising the hospital system took over.

The Fitzgerald Report

Since it was published in 1968, the Fitzgerald Report has provided a focus for discussion on the future development of the general hospital services. The report was prepared by a broadly representative group of consultants, under the chairmanship of the late Professor Patrick Fitzgerald, who were appointed as a consultative council by the minister, Sean Flanagan. The council made important recommendations in relation to administration (these are referred to on page 59), but the essential part of its task was to report on the organisation and location of these services:

> so as to secure, with due regard to the national resources, that the public is provided in a most effective way with the best possible services.

Having surveyed the present pattern of hospital services, the council concluded that radical changes were necessary,

123

involving a departure from many long-established concepts in organisation, staffing and operation. Its recommendations on administration, involving the creation of a central 'consultants establishment board', regional hospitals boards and hospital management committees, were aimed at achieving a re-organisation of the services involving closer co-ordination between the voluntary hospitals and the then local authority hospitals.

At the top level of the integrated structure, the council recommended that there should be four regional hospitals, two in Dublin and one each in Cork and Galway. Each of these would provide a general service for its own hinterland and more specialised services for a wider area. The council recommended that there should be general hospitals in nine other centres, each having at least 300 beds. The basic services provided in these would be general medicine, general surgery, obstetrics, gynaecology, pathology and radiology. In making this recommendation, the council pointed to the advantages of larger units (which allow for more specialisation), better staffing arrangements (because of there being a number of physicians and surgeons attached to each hospital) and the better equipment which would be possible in such hospitals.

Each of the general hospitals recommended by the council would serve a population of about 120,000 people. Only some of the county hospitals could be developed into these general hospitals and the functions of the others would change. The council envisaged that these would take patients of family doctors, who could continue to care for them while in hospital, and would be backed by diagnostic facilities and a comprehensive consultant out-patient organisation. These centres, the council pointed out, would have an important role in the care of long-stay geriatric patients. The district hospitals would also be used in conjunction with the family doctor service, but would not be regarded as having a role in the provision of acute care hospital services. In their development of these recommendations, the council set out detailed proposals for their application throughout the country.

The minister announced acceptance of the general principles of the Fitzgerald Report, but not of all the specific recommendations on the application of these principles throughout the country. The principles of the report are reflected in the developments which have taken place in Dublin and in many other areas since it was published, but its specific recommendations for the county hospitals were not accepted. It was clear that, whatever about the medical case for the proposals to concentrate the services, it was not politically practicable to consider their full implementation.

The hospital plan, 1975
After the health boards had taken over the regional, county and district hospitals from the local authorities, it seemed that specific county interests would be less prominent and that hospital planning should be on the basis of the new regions which were the functional areas of the boards. The boards were asked by the minister, Brendan Corish, to prepare proposals for development of their hospital systems on the basis of criteria for the size of hospitals and coverage of the population prepared by Comhairle na nOspideal. These proposals were endorsed by the minister and approved by the government in 1975 as a plan for future hospital development.

The 1975 plan proposed that the number of county hospitals giving full medical and surgical care would be reduced over time from 24 to 14 and that these would be expanded and developed by each health board to meet the needs of its area. The hospitals chosen for development were, in the north-west, Letterkenny and Sligo, in the north-east, Cavan and Dundalk, in the midlands, Portlaoise and Mullingar, in the south-east, Kilkenny, Waterford, Wexford and Cashel or Clonmel, in the south, Bantry and Tralee, in the mid-west, Ennis and in the west, Castlebar. This plan was the basis of most of the planning of hospital developments

125

since 1975 but it has been eroded over the years by decisions to retain almost all the county hospitals.

In Dublin, the plan allowed for six major general hospitals – the Beaumont, Mater and James Connolly Memorial hospitals[14] on the northside and the St Vincent's, St James's and Tallaght hospitals on the southside. Five of these hospitals are functioning now. The opening of Beaumont Hospital in November 1987 has led to the closure of St Laurence's and Jervis Street hospitals and the work of Mercer's, Sir Patrick Dun's, Dr Steevens and the Royal City of Dublin hospitals has been transferred to St James's Hospital. The Adelaide, the Meath and the National Children's Hospital continue to function pending the building of the Tallaght hospital.

The major general hospital in Cork is the health board's regional hospital. The four public voluntary hospitals in the city (the Mercy, the North Infirmary, the South Infirmary, the Victoria and the Eye, Ear and Throat) were federated in 1977 under the Cork Voluntary Hospitals Board,[15] with the objective of their ultimate amalgamation in a new hospital. The North Infirmary was closed in 1987.

PRIVATE HOSPITALS

Most of the private general hospitals are managed by religious orders. They are financed by charges made on patients which in the majority of cases are made by the Voluntary Health Insurance Board's schemes. Some contributions towards their costs are met by the health boards. Eight of the 17 private hospitals are in Dublin.

CAUSES OF STAY IN HOSPITAL

The Medico-Social Research Board initiated and maintained an ongoing survey on the medical conditions for which patients were kept in hospital (this project is now continued by the Health Research Board). The following were the main causes in 1983 shown as percentages of total discharges and the average durations of stay for each category:

Table 2: *Causes of stay in hospital*

Diagnosis	Cases as percentage of total	Average duration of stay (days)
Accidents, poisonings and violence	13.9	7.0
Diseases of respiratory system	11.3	10.4
Diseases of digestive system	11.2	7.8
Diseases of circulatory system	9.7	14.8
Symptoms and ill-defined conditions	9.6	5.9
Diseases of genito-urinary system	8.1	6.6
Special admissions and consultations	6.9	8.3
Neoplasms	5.6	13.5
Diseases of nervous system and sense organs	5.5	8.6

These conditions accounted for over 80 per cent of all admissions (excluding maternity, which was not covered by the survey).[16]

The five diagnostic categories listed in Table 3 accounted for almost 60 per cent of all bed-days in the hospitals surveyed.

Table 3: *Diagnostic categories*

circulatory system	15.9%
respiratory system	13.0%
accidents, poisoning and violence	10.8%
digestive system	9.7%
neoplasms	8.5%

PROVISION OF HOSPITAL SERVICES

The law on the provision of hospital in-patient and out-patient services by the health boards (and by the voluntary hospitals on their behalf) is contained in Chapter II of Part

IV of the Health Act, 1970 (as amended) and the regulations under that chapter of the act.

Eligibility for access to the services is described in Chapter five. Since May 1987, access has become subject to charges of £10 a day for inpatient care (up to a maximum of £100 in a year) and £10 for visits to out-patient clinics. Medical card holders and some other categories are exempt from these charges.[17]

In 1971, the liability for the cost of hospital services arising from road accidents was placed on the person causing the injury (where identified). The provision in the regulations on this was contested in court and, on an appeal to the Supreme Court, was found *ultra vires*. However, this liability was restored under the Health (Amendment) Act, 1986.

COMPARISON WITH OTHER EC MEMBER STATES

A study carried out for the year 1976 compared hospital resources and their use in the EC[18]:

Table 4: *Use of hospital resources in the EC(9)*

Country	Beds per 1,000 population	Admissions per 1,000 population
Belgium	6.4	n.a.
Denmark	6.4	172
France	8.1	168
Federal Republic of Germany	10.0	163
Ireland	**5.8**	**162**
Italy	8.6	171
Luxembourg	7.1	119
Netherlands	5.2	104
United Kingdom	8.7	115

These figures relate to general hospitals only. They would indicate that the hospital system in Ireland in 1976 was not overblown relative to the other EC countries. The throughput of patients in Irish hospitals (28 per bed in that year) was the highest in the EC. One must be careful, however, in making comparisons in this field. Definitions of what is a hospital can vary between countries.

NOTES ON CHAPTER ELEVEN

1. The sources of the figures in this paragraph are tables 1 (page 52) and G 13 (page 73) in Health Statistics, 1986 (Department of Health), published by the Stationery Office.
2. Ibid. table G 2
3. Ibid. table 2, page 53
4. Ibid. table 3, page 53
5. Ibid. table 4, page 54 (there were five fever hospitals up to 1984. The New Ross hospital was closed in April, 1985)
6. Outline of the Future Hospital System – Report of the Consultative Council on the General Hospital Services, 1968 (Prl 154)
7. Table G 7, Health Statistics 1981 and Health Statistics 1986 (comparative figures for years before 1979 are not available)
8. Health Statistics, 1986, table G 7
9. Ibid. table G 7
10. Ibid. table G 8
11. See the Blood Transfusion Board (Establishment) Order 1965 (S.I. 78 of 1965)
12. See the Hospital Sterile Supplies Board (Establishment) Order 1965 (S.I. 1 of 1965) and an amending order of the same year (S.I. 157 of 1965)
13. Section 57 of the Health Act, 1970
14. The James Connolly Memorial Hospital, originally a major sanatorium, became a general hospital administered by a board set up in 1971 under the Health (Corporate Bodies) Act, 1961. In 1987, its administration was transferred back to the Eastern Health Board.
15. See the Cork Voluntary Hospitals Board (Establishment) Order 1977 (S.I. 290 of 1977)
16. Health Statistics, 1986, table G 10
17. These charges are imposed by the Health (In-patient Charges) Regulations 1987 (S.I. 116 of 1987) and the Health Services (Out-patient Charges) Regulations, 1987 (S.I. 115 of 1987). To allow the latter regulations to be made, section 56(3) of the Health Act, 1970 was amended by the Health (Amendment) Act, 1987
18. Based on Table G 11, Health Statistics, 1985

CHAPTER TWELVE

Information for planning

Information on the size of the population, on birth, death and marriage rates and on the numbers affected by different diseases and injuries is vital to the organisation of the health services. This information is necessary in identifying problems, in designing services, in deciding on priorities in development and in evaluating the results of action taken. The reports prepared by the Central Statistics Office (CSO) on the periodic censuses of population[1] form the basis for statistical information on the health services. These give information to the department and to the health boards on the numbers for whom health services must be designed. To build on this, the department and other agencies analyse information specifically relating to health and the health services.

BIRTHS, DEATHS AND MARRIAGES

Under the Minister for Health, an tArd Chlaraitheoir (the Registrar-General) has the responsibility for organising the registration of births, deaths and marriages. He operates through local registrars who come under the general supervision of the health boards. As well as the basic data needed for registration, further detailed information relating to births and deaths is compiled. From this, annual reports on vital statistics are published by the minister, with the co-operation of the CSO.[2] The detailed operation of this system is described in Appendix F.

The registration system is concerned with the causes of death but not with the incidence of disease in living persons.

The only formal requirements for providing such information relate to the notification of infectious diseases referred to in chapter six.

RESEARCH

The Medical Research Council
The Medical Research Council was incorporated as a limited liability company in 1937, with the object of organising and carrying out research in medicine. The council had nine members, made up of eight nominees of the universities and other medical licensing bodies and a chairman appointed by the minister. The council administered funds made available to it by the minister and from other sources.

The council's primary concern was with basic research on the causes of and cures for diseases and most of its funds were devoted to giving grants for projects in these fields. It was not part of the council's function to conduct widespread projects on morbidity or on the operation of the health services.

The Medico-Social Research Board
To extend work on morbidity and social research, the Medico-Social Research Board was established in 1965.[3] Its functions were to organise and administer surveys and statistical research in relation to the incidence of human diseases, injuries, deformities and defects, and the operation of the health services. The board had fourteen members who were appointed by the minister.

The board conducted a continuing survey in relation to in-patients in general hospitals. The hospitals were asked to complete statistical summaries for all patients and to send them to the board, which had the data processed. The information gleaned from this survey includes a diagnostic index for each of the participating hospitals and for each participating consultant (on request), and national statistics, showing discharges from hospitals by reference to diagnosis and duration of stay. Some results from this survey are shown on page 127.

A national psychiatric in-patient reporting system was also operated by the board and studies were undertaken by it on specific psychiatric subjects. It also conducted a census of mentally handicapped in the community and in institutions. Follow-up studies on the causes of mental handicap and its prevalence were undertaken. Among other projects conducted by the board were a study of peri-natal and child mortality and morbidity in Ireland, studies on the incidence of ischaemic heart disease and strokes (both of these were carried out in collaboration with the World Health Organisation), a study on air pollution (as part of EC studies on environmental control) and studies on the incidence of drug abuse. The board was co-sponsor, with the Irish Heart Foundation, of the Kilkenny Health Project.

The Health Research Board
In 1986, the functions of the Medical Research Council and the Medico-Social Research Board were taken over by the Health Research Board.[4] Its membership consists of sixteen persons appointed by the minister, half of them being nominated conjointly by the teaching bodies formerly involved in the Medical Research Council. The term of office of members is five years. The first chairman of the new board was appointed by the minister but subsequent chairmen will be elected by the members of the board.

The functions of the new board relate to medical research and medico-social research. The board will also have a role in 'health services research', meaning 'research into the organisation, management, delivery and financing of health and personal social services.'

DIGESTS OF HEALTH STATISTICS

Each year the planning unit of the Department of Health

issues *Health Statistics,* which gives a digest of statistical
material relevant to the health services. It covers population
and vital statistics, each of the health programmes referred
to in earlier chapters, manpower, finance and eligibility.[5]

NOTES ON CHAPTER TWELVE

1. Published by the Stationery Office, Dublin
2. Published by the Stationery Office, Dublin
3. Under the Medico-Social Research Board (Establishment) Order, 1965
   (S.I. 80 of 1965), which was amended by another order in 1974 (S.I.
   169 of 1965)
4. Set up under the Health Research Board (Establishment) Order, 1986
   (S.I. 279 of 1965)
5. Published by the Stationery Office, Dublin

CHAPTER THIRTEEN

Organisation

The power to decide what health services there will be and how they will be administered does not reside in any one person or institution. Basically, of course, the civil authority for the provision of the services comes from the legislature. It flows mainly through the Minister for Health but, in substantial volume, it passes on to the several functional bodies concerned in the provision of the services. They in their turn, together with special advisory bodies, may influence the course of this flow – generally in an indirect fashion through the minister. Figure 1 below illustrates the administration.

Figure 1: *Administration of the Health Services*

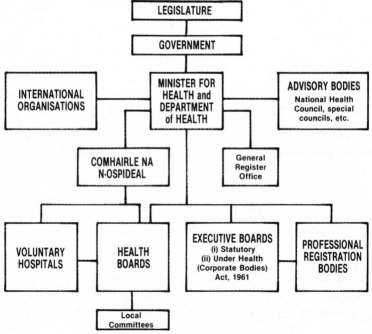

134

CENTRAL ADMINISTRATION

The legislature.
The legal basis for the health services is contained in the acts passed by the Dail and Seanad, and the actions of all the other organs of administration must conform with those acts. In general, the acts governing the provision of the health services (and notably the Health Acts of 1947, 1953 and 1970) do not lay down in detail how the services will operate but leave this to regulations made by the minister, to guidelines and directives issued by his department and to the decisions of the health boards and other executive agencies.

The minister, in preparing regulations, cannot do anything which the parent act does not provide for and the content of regulations is subject to control by the legislature. In a few instances (such as the regulations on the establishment and constitution of the health boards), a draft must be approved by the Dail and Seanad before the regulations are made. Where this does not apply the regulations must be presented to both houses after they are made and either house may, by resolution, annul them within a specified period. This control is one which is unlikely to be used but its existence could be a curb on an unreasonable minister.

The Dail also exercises a control on the actions of the minister by its debates on the annual estimates for the Department of Health. In addition, members of the Dail have the right to ask questions of the minister on the operation of the services and, if they wish, to initiate a fuller discussion if they think the reply is unsatisfactory. The Dail's committees on public accounts and on public expenditure exercise a continuing surveillance on public expenditure on the health services.[1]

The government.
As in the case of the other branches of the public services, decisions on the initiation of health legislation rests with the government. So do other major decisions on health policy.

These are normally taken on the basis of submissions made by the Minister for Health and, before any decision is taken by the government, other ministers concerned will have considered the proposal from their point of view.

The Minister for Health and his department
Broadly, the role of the Minister for Health is to see that the health care system operates to the best effect and in accordance with legislation and government policy. He also initiates and pursues policies to change the system and the working of it when he thinks this is for the public good. The minister has wide powers relating to the making of statutory regulations and orders and to the general supervision of the activities of the health boards and other executive agencies in the provision of health services. As the co-ordinating and supervising authority for the services, the minister's functions range from approving the general pattern to control of the method of appointment, the remuneration and the conditions of service of health personnel. The minister does not have any power to give directions on the eligibility of individual persons for health services or on how the services are to be made available to individuals. Such decisions are left to the subordinate agencies.

The transfer of administration to the eight health boards in 1971 led to a review of the methods of supervision of the services by the minister. More emphasis was placed on control by way of general guidelines and directives, coupled with budgetary controls, in place of many of the individual approvals called for in the past. The Health Act, 1970 and the regulations made under it were designed to permit this.

The statutory powers are vested in the minister. Decisions on the use of these powers are his responsibility, but, in accordance with the Ministers and Secretaries Acts, the Department of Health is there to deal with the 'departmental administration' relative to the minister's functions. This 'departmental administration' is, in fact, the taking of whatever action is necessary (and permitted by law) to execute the decisions on policy made by the minister. The department also provides information and advice to the minister on matters arising for his decision.

The head of the department is the secretary, who has overall administrative control of the department and has the main responsibility for seeing that the minister's policies are implemented. The secretary is also charged personally with the responsibility for ensuring that all payments made from the department's vote are legally and properly made for purposes covered by the vote. He must, therefore, be especially careful to warn the minister if he thinks that any expenditure which the latter directs is not covered by the Vote for Health.

The organisation of the Department of Health follows the principles set out in the Report of the Public Services Organisation Review Group (see page 55). The report proposed that each department should be re-arranged so as to separate policy-making from executive functions. The Department of Health was the first to be re-organised on this basis.

The policy-making component in a department restructured in this way is called the aireacht and, in accordance with the PSORG report, it is made up of 'staff' units and 'line' divisions. The staff units are for planning, finance, organisation and personnel. In addition, because of the strong professional input required in the Department of Health, the chief medical officer and other professional staff retain a separate status within the aireacht. The 'line' divisions of the aireacht are in three groups, one for community health services, one for welfare services and one for general hospital services.

The Department of Health's main role has been in the field of policy-making; the execution of policies in the health services is left almost entirely to the outside agencies described later in this chapter. The only executive units within the department are the office of the Registrar-General for Births, Deaths and Marriages, the Hospital Planning Office (which

co-operates with executive agencies in the design and building
of hospitals) and a section dealing with the superannuation
scheme for voluntary hospitals.

The PSORG Report envisaged that in each aireacht a
management advisory committee should be constituted to
advise the secretary in the formulation of proposals for the
minister. The management advisory committee in the
Department of Health consists of the secretary, the chief
medical officer and the assistant secretaries. Heads of other
units and other members of the professional staff may also
be asked to attend meetings of the committee.[2]

Advisory bodies
The Minister for Health and the department have many
sources of advice. On broad policy issues, there is, of course,
a steady stream of opinion from parliamentary debates and,
on more detailed points, the minister in the normal course of
his political activity will see a reflection of public opinion in
what is said and written to him. There are also many
contacts, of different degrees of formality, between the
minister and departmental officers, representative members
of the health professions and those involved in health board
administration. Advice is available on a more institutionalised
basis from a number of bodies.

The National Health Council is the general statutory
advisory body on the health services. Its function is 'to advise
the minister on such general matters affecting or incidental
to the health of the people as may be referred to them by
the minister and on such other general matters (other than
conditions of employment of officers and servants and the
amount of payment of grants and allowances) relating to the
operation of the health services as they think fit'. The council
is appointed by the minister but at least half of the members
must be 'nominated by bodies representative of the medical
and ancillary professions and of persons concerned with the
management of voluntary hospitals'. The selection of the
other members of the council rests with the minister but it
has been the practice to include persons involved in other

bodies concerned with health questions, such as the trade unions. The members of the council serve for two years.

The National Health Council appoints its own chairman and regulates its own procedure but, if it wishes to meet more than three times in any quarter, it musk seek the consent of the minister. An officer of the department acts as secretary to the council. Its meetings are held in private.

The minister is required to seek the council's advice before he makes regulations under the Health Acts or the Mental Treatment Acts. If, because of urgency, the minister cannot arrange this before he makes the regulations, he is obliged to ask for the council's advice on them after they have been made. Advising on regulations, however, forms only part of the council's work. It has concerned itself with and reported on practically all the major developments in the health services which have been considered since it was reconstituted in its present form in 1954. The council presents an annual report to the minister who is obliged to publish it, with comments if deemed necessary.[3]

There is a host of specialist advisory bodies. These are of two kinds, standing statutory bodies and special bodies which are set up from time to time to advise on specific problems. The former group includes Comhairle na nOspideal, the Health Research Board, the National Drugs Advisory Board and the statutory professional registration bodies (described in chapter fourteen). There have been many special advisory bodies in the health field. The constitution of such a body can range from a formal commission of enquiry (as in the case of the commission on mental illness set up in 1964), through a consultative council set up by statutory instrument, to an informal working party. Practically all aspects of the health services have at one time or another been covered by investigations by bodies such as these. The reports of various advisory bodies which influenced health policy are included in the bibliography on page 276.

Comhairle na nOspideal.
As well as being an advisory body Comhairle na nOspideal

has a statutory executive role in regulating the numbers and types of consultant appointments in hospitals taking patients under the Health Acts and in specifying qualifications for the appointment of consultants.

The comhairle was established under section 41 of the Health Act, 1970. At least half of its members must be 'registered medical practitioners engaged in a consultant capacity in the provision of hospital services'. It has twenty-seven members, of whom at least fourteen are in this category. The other appointees include officers of the Department of Health and persons involved in voluntary hospitals and in the health boards. The chairman and vice-chairman of the comhairle are selected by the minister from amongst the members. The comhairle has authority to establish committees and has used this authority widely.[4]

LOCAL EXECUTIVE BODIES

Health boards
The organs of central administration mentioned above are mainly concerned with broad questions of health policy, of the scope of the services and of how they should be organised. The main burden of work in operating the services decreed by these central authorities is laid on the health boards.

Section 4(1) of the Health Act, 1970, provided:

For the administration of health services in the State, the Minister shall, after consultation with the Minister for Local Government, by regulations establish such number of boards (to be known and in this Act referred to as health boards) as may appear to him to be appropriate, and by such regulations shall specify the title and define the functional area of each health board so established and, subject to sub-section (2), shall specify the membership of each health board

140

Section 4 (2) specified in broad terms the constitution of each health board. The majority of the members must be appointed by the local county councils and county borough corporations (and, in the case of the Eastern Health Board, the Corporation of Dun Laoghaire) and the remainder of the membership must include persons elected by medical practitioners and members of ancillary professions. Under section 4 (4), consultations with the county councils and other nominating local authorities were required before regulations were made under the section.

Each health board set up under the act is a body corporate, with the usual authority to hold and dispose of land, etc. The act contains rules relating to the membership and meetings of the boards and provisions allowing them to set up committees (to which functions may be delegated), to act jointly in providing services (including, if necessary, the establishment of a joint body) and to co-operate with local authorities. The boards can also enter into arrangements with other bodies, such as voluntary hospitals, to provide services on their behalf.[5]

Eight such boards were set up in 1970.[6] The map and table on pages 142–3 set out the areas served by these boards and the constitution of each of them.

In designing this structure, a number of factors were taken into account. Inter-county arrangements for other services were borne in mind, in particular the regions for local government planning and development (in fact, for health purposes only Roscommon and Meath are in combinations with other counties which are different from the local government combinations). Regard was also had to the desirability of not combining too many counties in any one board, of not allowing the population to be served to be much below 200,000 persons in any case, and of not having any board covering too extensive an area. It was not, however, by using any exact formula that the decision was taken to have eight boards. This result of detailed discussions and consideration was necessarily a compromise based on commonsense rather than on science.

Health Board areas and headquarters

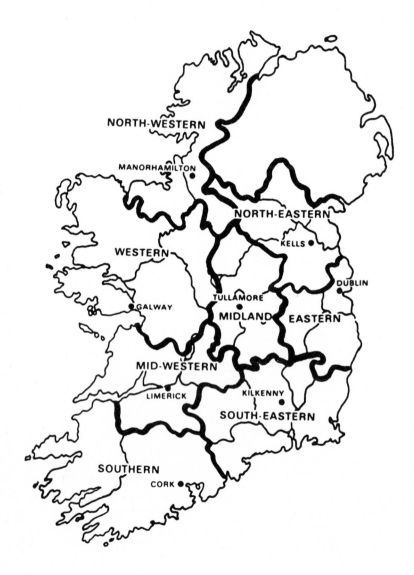

NORTH-WESTERN

MANORHAMILTON •

NORTH-EASTERN

KELLS •

WESTERN

DUBLIN

GALWAY •

TULLAMORE •

MIDLAND

EASTERN

MID-WESTERN

LIMERICK •

KILKENNY •

SOUTH-EASTERN

SOUTHERN

CORK •

Table 1: *Health Boards, membership*

Title of Board	Functional area	Population (1981)	local authority members	medical practitioners	dentists	pharmacists	general nurses	psychiatric nurses	ministerial nominees	total
Eastern Health Board	Dublin City and County, Counties, Kildare and Wicklow (1,800 sq. miles)	1,195,000	19	9	1	1	1	1	3	35
Midland Health Board	Counties Laois, Longford, Offaly and Westmeath (2,250 sq. miles)	202,000	16	7	1	1	1	1	3	30
Mid-Western Health Board	Counties Clare, Limerick City and County, County Tipperary (N.R.) (3,040 sq. miles)	308,000	15	6	1	1	1	1	3	28
North-Eastern Health Board	Counties Cavan, Louth, Meath, Monaghan (1,950 sq. miles)	289,000	16	7	1	1	1	1	3	30
North-Western Health Board	Counties Donegal, Leitrim and Sligo (2,600 sq. miles)	208,000	14	6	1	1	1	1	3	27
South-Eastern Health Board	Counties Carlow, Kilkenny, Tipperary (S.R.), County and City of Waterford and County Wexford (6,630 sq. miles)	375,000	16	8	1	1	1	1	3	31
Southern Health Board	County and City of Cork and County Kerry (4,700 sq. miles)	525,000	18	8	1	1	1	1	3	33
Western Health Board	Counties Galway, Mayo and Roscommon (5,020 sq. miles)	341,000	15	7	1	1	1	1	3	29

143

Local committees
Local committees, primarily advisory, are provided for by section 7 of the 1970 Act. In the case of most counties, there is one local committee for the county. Local councillors are in a majority in the membership of these committees. The constitution for a county advisory committee is:

1. three councillors from each electoral area (in those local authorities where there are only four electoral areas, the council appoints three further councillors to ensure a local authority majority),

2. the county manager (or his nominee),

3. the director of community care,

4. the chief psychiatrist (or another senior psychiatrist),

5. a consultant from a general hospital,

6. two other doctors elected by the profession,

7. the superintendent community welfare officer,

8. a psychiatric nurse,

9. a public health nurse,

10. a dentist,

11. a pharmacist,

12. two other persons, not being councillors, who are associated with voluntary organisations in the sphere of social services.

Meetings of a local committee are attended by the chief executive officer or another senior officer of the health board. The general pattern for the constitution of local committees is varied for the four areas which include county boroughs.[7]

Management in health boards
Each health board is required to have 'a person who shall

be called and shall act as the chief executive officer to the board'. The provisions in the 1970 Act on the functions of the chief executive officer make an interesting departure from those in the County Management Acts which governed the management of the services under the former local administration. The management acts gave to the county manager the statutory responsibility for practically all the functions of the county council, although in performing them he was subject to restrictions and directions by the council. Under the 1970 Act only a limited range of decisions, mainly relating to eligibility of individuals for services and personnel matters,are reserved to the chief executive officer of a health board. Outside of these matters he and the other officers of the board are specifically required to 'act in accordance with such decisions and directions (whether of a general or a particular nature) as are conveyed to or through the chief executive officer by the board, and in accordance with any such decisions and directions so conveyed of a committee to which functions have been delegated by the board'. The chief executive officer or another officer acting in accordance with such a direction, is regarded as acting on behalf of the board.[8]

In fact, the health boards have recognised the need to delegate the day-to-day management of the services on a considerable scale to their chief executive officers, while retaining ultimate control in their own hands.

The management team

For management purposes, the work of a health board is in three broad divisions covering respectively community care services, general hospital services and 'special' hospital services (these being in the main the hospital services for the mentally ill and the mentally handicapped). Each of these divisions is in the charge of a programme manager. In the larger boards there is a separate programme manager for each of the three divisions, while in each of the smaller boards (the midland, north-eastern and north-western boards), there are only two programme managers, one of whom covers both of the hospital programmes. In addition, there are 'functional' officers in charge of finance, personnel and planning (in the case of the smaller boards, finance and planning are combined under one officer). This group of officers, under the chief executive officer, form the 'management team' for the health board.

Members of the management team have their own specific responsibilities, but they are expected to act together as a group in evolving policy and advising the board on the future lines of development. Figure 2 below illustrates the management structure for the larger boards.

Figure 2: *Health Board management structure*

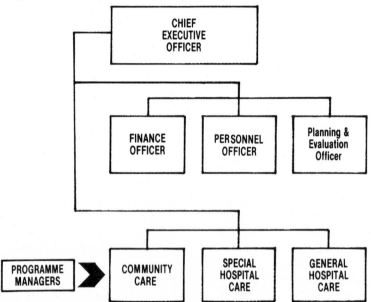

Community care staff

The community care division in a health board covers the preventive health services, the general practitioner services and other domiciliary services, dental and public health nursing services and the community welfare programme. For the administration of community care, each health board's area is divided into sub-areas which in rural areas generally coincide with the counties. The services in the community are co-ordinated by the directors of community care. They are responsible to the programme manager for the operation of this range of services. Figure 3 below illustrates the organisation of the community care programme. The positions on this chart do not necessarily indicate the relative status of the officers shown.

Figure 3: *Community Care organisation*

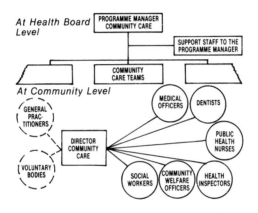

Organisation for general hospitals

The programme manager, general hospital care, has responsibility for planning general hospital services for the population served by the health board. Unlike the programme manager for community care, he will not have under him a county or community organisation, but has a small support staff. Each of the major hospitals of a health board has a resident hospital administrator and smaller hospitals may be grouped for this purpose under one administrator. Health boards are also recommended to establish executive committees for the larger and more complex institutions, with membership and functions so designed as to draw the consultants and other staff in the hospitals into their administration.

Special hospital programme staff
Under the programme manager, the officers directing the psychiatric service are the chief psychiatrists and, in larger urban areas, clinical directors for subdivisions of the area. Because the services for the mentally handicapped are provided mainly in voluntary institutions, most health boards have no special directorate for this service.

OTHER EXECUTIVE BODIES

Not all the executive work in relation to the health services is suited to local administration. For those parts of it not so suited, the practice has evolved of setting up special central executive agencies. Some of these were set up by statute and others were formerly set up by arranging for the establishment of a company under the Companies Acts. Among the former, the most noteworthy example is the Voluntary Health Insurance Board; the latter included the Medical Research Council, which was established in 1937, and bodies to administer the blood transfusion service and the mass radiography service.

The Health (Corporate Bodies) Act, 1961 brought in a new, more easily used, procedure for setting up such executive bodies. The minister is authorised to set up a corporate body to administer a health service by an order under the act. Such an order, which is liable to annulment by either house of the Oireachtas, specifies the constitution and functions of the body established and includes provision for the appointment of staff, etc. This act has over the years been used to set up many new executive agencies, including the National Drugs Advisory Board and the Health Education Bureau, as well as boards for a number of hospitals. The most recent use of this act was in the establishment in 1986 of the Health Research Board which has replaced the Medical

Research Council and the Medico-Social Research Board
(see page 132).

A provision of the 1961 act allowed a limited liability
company established earlier as an executive body for the
health services to be transformed into a body under the new
act. The Blood Transfusion Service Board and the National
Rehabilitation Board are among the bodies which were so
transformed.

There is power to authorise the health boards as a group,
(or two or more of them) to act through a specially
established joint board.[9] This provision is the basis for the
General Medical Services (Payments) Board, the central
bureau for paying doctors and pharmacists under the general
medical service.

While the voluntary hospitals are not executive bodies
within the sphere of public administration like those referred
to above, an account of the executive agencies in the health
services would be incomplete without referring to those
hospitals. The voluntary hospitals participate in a large way
in providing services for the public authorities. A number of
other associations and agencies co-operate with the public
authorities in the provision of the health services. Included
among these are councils or associations for specific diseases
or conditions, and bodies concerned in the organisation of
social services.

INTERNATIONAL HEALTH ORGANISATIONS

Ireland plays its part in a number of inter-governmental
health bodies and its services benefit from participation in
the work of these bodies through information obtained on
what is done elsewhere, through reports of international
technical work and through sending her nationals abroad on
study tours organised by these bodies.

The World Health Organisation
The World Health Organisation (WHO) is paramount

among the international health bodies. This organisation was founded in 1948 as a specialised agency of the United Nations Organisation and took over the work of the International Office of Public Health of the League of Nations. The constitution of the organisation lists its functions,[10] the more important ones being: to act as the directing and co-ordinating authority on international health work, to assist governments, upon request, in strengthening health services and to furnish technical assistance and, in emergencies, necessary aid.

The legislative organ of WHO is the annual assembly. This is attended by representatives of the 164 member states of the organisation. At the assembly, the budget is approved, international regulations are made and questions of general interest are debated. The responsibility for seeing that the decisions of the assembly are carried out is vested in the executive board of the organisation, which is made up of persons nominated by thirty of the member states. The staff of WHO is headed by the director-general. It is his responsibility to propose the budget for submission by the executive board to the assembly and to see to the execution of the decisions of the assembly and the board. The headquarters of the organisation is in Geneva. Its total budget for 1987 was £152 million.

The execution of the policies of WHO is to a great extent delegated to subsidiary regional organisations. This country is concerned with the European Regional Office, with headquarters in Copenhagen. The regional organisations have their own staffs and work in conjunction with regional committees made up of representatives of the member states of the region.

The organisation has power to make regulations binding on its members. The most important of these are the International Sanitary Regulations which govern the restrictions which may be imposed on the movements of international traffic to prevent the spread of infectious diseases, and the International Regulations on Health Statistics which provide a standardised list of diseases and causes of death. The more

highly-developed members of WHO benefit through fellowships and seminars organised by the regional organisations.
A number of fellowships are granted each year to each
member of the region and the individual states are accorded
a wide discretion in choosing the fellows and the subjects of
study. The arrangements for the course of study in each case
are made by the organisation, whose wide experience is very
valuable in this respect. A wide variety of studies has been
pursued by Irish fellows under this scheme.

The Council of Europe
The Council of Europe is an organisation of twenty-one
European states (Austria, Belgium, Cyprus, Denmark, France,
the Federal Republic of Germany, Greece, Iceland, Ireland,
Italy, Liechtenstein, Luxembourg, Malta, Netherlands,
Norway, Portugal, Spain, Sweden, Switzerland, Turkey and
the United Kingdom), which was established in 1949. Its
aim is 'to achieve a greater unity between its members for
the purpose of safeguarding and realising the ideals and
principles which are their common heritage and facilitating
their economic and social progress'. Health questions are not,
of course, the primary concern of the Council of Europe but
its programme includes the encouragement of its members to
co-operate with each other in providing health services and
to co-ordinate their health programmes. In this it avoids
duplicating the work of WHO, with which it maintains
liaison. Representatives of the health organisations of the
member states of the council meet twice yearly in Strasbourg.
Among steps towards co-ordinating their health services are
the establishment of direct contacts between the administrations and examination of the technical and administrative
difficulties in the way of mutual aid in providing health
services, both normally and in times of disasters. The council
also provides fellowships for members of the medical and
paramedical professions and of the health services, so that
they can become conversant with new techniques practised
in European countries and can participate in studies and
research of common European interest. Several of these

fellowships have been awarded to candidates from Ireland.

Eleven of the member states of the Council of Europe-Austria, Belgium, Denmark, France, the Federal Republic of Germany, Ireland, Italy, Luxembourg, the Netherlands, Switzerland and the United Kingdom – have, under the aegis of the council, entered into a 'partial agreement' to co-operate in certain public health matters. This deals, in particular, with arrangements for health control of sea and air travel, with health controls on foodstuffs and with controls on poisonous substances in agriculture.

The European Community (EC)
The European Economic Community was set up in 1958 under the Treaty of Rome. The present members of the Community are Belgium, Denmark, France, the Federal Republic of Germany, Greece, Ireland, Italy, Luxembourg, the Netherlands, Portugal, Spain, and the United Kingdom. While the Treaty of Rome contains little in the way of specific provisions on health services, the activities of the community include a number of matters relating to the health services and these involve certain obligations for this country.

It is an aim of the Treaty of Rome to allow nationals of each of the member states of the community freedom to work in other member states and the commission, the executive of the community, has the duty to issue directives to bring about this freedom. These directives include requirements for mutual recognition of professional qualifications and registrations between the member states. They are discussed in chapter fourteen.

Also in furtherance of the aim of having free movement of workers, the community has made regulations for migrant workers, so that they can carry entitlement to social services from one country to another, both for themselves and their dependants. As far as health services are concerned, this means that, when a person covered by the social security system of another EC country needs urgent medical care when temporarily in Ireland, our health authorities have an obligation to provide it, the cost being charged to the person's home social security system. It also means that if a person who has a social security pension from the system in one EC country goes to live in another EC country, the health authorities in the latter may charge the cost of health care provided for him to the country where he was insured. Under these regulations, the Department of Health gets a considerable net income from other EC countries (mainly the United Kingdom).[11]

Other instruments of the EC aim to remove causes of distortion in competition and are designed to introduce standardisation in the controls on the manufacture and sale of a number of products. The Department of Health is involved in this respect as far as quality control of pharmaceutical products and the directives governing additives and colouring matters in food are concerned.

While entry into the EC has affected our health services in a number of ways, there is nothing in the Treaty of Rome or in the activities of the community up to the present which would suggest that a common health care system will be designed for the members.

Other inter-governmental organisations
Some other international organisations are concerned with health questions. The United Nations Organisation (UNO) is responsible for the administration of the conventions on traffic in dangerous drugs and one of its specialised agencies, the Food and Agriculture Organisation (FAO), has functions in connection with nutrition and food standards. The International Labour Office (ILO) concerns itself with such matters as standards for social security (including eligibility for health services), medical examination of various classes of workers and the rehabilitation of the disabled. The International Civil Aviation Organisation (ICAO) which regulates international air traffic, is concerned with the extent of the health precautions required for such traffic under WHO regulations. The International Atomic Energy Agency deals with health protection in the field of nuclear energy.

Other international bodies

As well as these bodies representative of governments, there are a large number of international health organisations which are directly representative of professional or specialised interests in countries throughout the world. The World Medical Association, for example, is representative of the medical associations of most countries. In addition to organising its own meetings at which professional subjects are discussed, the association holds a watching brief on behalf of the medical profession at the assemblies of WHO. The International Hospital Federation is another example of these bodies. Its members are bodies interested in hospital construction and hospital services.

NOTES ON CHAPTER THIRTEEN

1. The working of the legislature is described in *The Houses of the Oireachtas* by J.C. Smyth, Institute of Public Administration, fourth edition 1979
2. This structure follows a report of a task force, Restructuring the Department of Health: the Separation of Policy and Execution, 1974 (Prl 3445)
3. See section 98 of the Health Act, 1947, as amended by section 41 of the Health Act, 1953
4. The regulation under section 41 are the Health (Hospital Bodies) Regulations 1972 (S.I. 164 of 1972)
5. See section 5, 8 to 11, 25 and 26 and the Second Schedule to the 1970 act. The Health Boards (Election of Members) Regulations, 1972 (S.I. 60 of 1977) are also relevant
6. Under the Health Boards Regulations, 1970 (S.I. 170 of 1970)
7. The Health (Local Committees) Regulations, 1972 (S.I. 31 of 1972)
8. Section 17 of the 1970 act.
9. Section 11 of the Health Act, 1970
10. This, and other WHO publications may be purchased through the Government Publications Sale Office
11. £21.4 million in 1985

CHAPTER FOURTEEN

Personnel

Health services are for the giving of care by persons to persons. The 'health care industry' is, therefore, highly labour intensive. The public sector in 1984 employed about 58,000 persons (including doctors and pharmacists engaged under contract in the general medical service). There is a much smaller number in the purely private sector, mainly those working in hospitals and homes and in private practice in the community. Remuneration for those working in the public health services accounts for about 67 per cent of the expenditure on those services.

THE HEALTH PROFESSIONS

Medical practitioners

The medical profession is governed by the Medical Council which was established by the Medical Practitioners Act, 1978, to replace the body set up in 1927 which is referred to on page 28. There are twenty-five members on the new council, made up of five appointed by the authorities of the undergraduate medical schools, six appointed to represent medical and surgical specialties, psychiatry and general practice, ten registered medical practitioners elected by the profession and four other persons appointed by the minister (at least three of these being non-doctors representing the interests of the general public). The members have a five-year term of office. The principal functions of the council relate to:

1. the general registration of medical practitioners and the maintenance of a register of medical specialists,
2. standards of education and training at undergraduate and post-graduate levels,
3. questions of professional misconduct or fitness to practise, and
4. the operation of EC directives relating to the practice of medicine.

The council is financed out of 'funds at the disposal of the council', mainly derived from registration and retention fees and fees for other services.

The most important duty of the council is to keep the General Register of Medical Practitioners. Each student obtaining any of the approved primary qualifications is entitled to be provisionally registered and then, after completing a year's hospital service as an intern, to become fully registered. A national of another member state of the EC qualified in medicine in his home country is entitled to be registered in the Irish register (Irish nationals are similarly entitled to be included in the registers of the other member states).[1] A person qualified in medicine in a non-EC country may be given full registration in Ireland if the Medical Council is satisfied as to the standard of his qualifications.[2]

Doctors from a number of foreign states, after qualification, are employed in Irish hospitals to gain experience. To facilitate this practice a system of temporary registration is provided for.[3] This permits the council to register any foreign graduate whose qualifications are regarded as adequate. Temporary registration is limited to whatever period the council fixes in each case and lapses in any event when the foreign graduate is no longer employed in the hospital. The aggregate of periods of temporary registration which the council is empowered to grant for any individual may not exceed five years.

Only registered medical practitioners are qualified by law to sign medical certificates.[4] The controls on drugs and medical preparations mentioned in chapter six prohibit the prescription or supply of a wide range of these by unregistered persons. As long as these restrictions are not breached, unregistered persons are not prevented from giving medical or surgical advice or treatment, but would be liable to penalties if they represented themselves as being registered. Furthermore, an unregistered person would not be entitled to sue for fees or charges.

The Medical Council has the duty of satisfying itself that the standard of knowledge required at examinations held by the medical schools is adequate. In the event of the council deciding that a medical school was no longer adequate there is a procedure whereby the minister on the recommendation of the council can withdraw recognition. The council also must satisfy itself that clinical training and experience provided during the 'intern year' is of an appropriate standard. It also has the duty to ensure that standards of postgraduate education and training provided by bodies recognised by it for medical specialist training are adequate and for ensuring that minimum EC requirements in this regard are met.

The Postgraduate Medical and Dental Board was also set up under the 1978 act. Its members come mainly from the bodies involved in postgraduate medical education and it is financed by a state grant. Its main functions are:

1. to promote the development of postgraduate medical and dental education and training and to co-ordinate such developments;
2. to advise the Minister for Health on the development and co-ordination of such training;
3. to provide career guidance for registered medical practitioners and dentists.

This board complements the role of the Medical Council by overseeing the organisation of specialist training. It has recognised ten main Irish professional training bodies as fulfilling major roles in programmed postgraduate training in various specialties. Under the aegis of these bodies, training posts are approved within hospitals, in general practice and in community medicine.

There are five undergraduate medical schools in Ireland – those in the Royal College of Surgeons (which issues qualifications jointly with the Royal College of Physicians), the University of Dublin (Trinity College) and the University Colleges in Dublin, Cork and Galway. Apart from the College of Surgeons, these schools are dependent mainly on state finance, channelled through the Higher Education Authority. Most of the students in the College of Surgeons come from abroad but only a small proportion of students in the other colleges are foreign. The total annual intake of students in recent years has been about 430.[5]

It is estimated that there are about 5,200 medical practitioners in Ireland. Some 4,300 (83%) of these are engaged in the public service (mainly the health boards and the voluntary hospitals). The number in the civil service, the army and other sectors is about 80. The percentages of the total in the public service engaged in the different services are shown in Figure 1 below.[6]

Figure 1: *Medical practitioners in the public service*

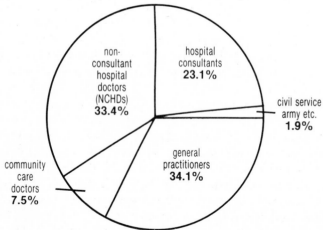

The nine hundred or so estimated as being engaged entirely

in private practice would include general practitioners who are outside the general medical service, consultants and other doctors in private hospitals and clinics, industrial medical officers and those wholetime in research.

Table 1 below shows the numbers of doctors per 100,000 population for each member state of the EC in 1976 and 1982:[7]

Table 1: *Doctors in the EC (9) (per 100,000)*

	1976	1982
Belgium	204	252
Denmark	195	237
France	163	263
Federal Republic of Germany	199	289
Ireland	**120**	**147**
Italy	225	322
Luxembourg	113	165
Netherlands	166	201
United Kingdom	138	161

Dentists

Under the Dentists Act, 1985, a new body, the Dental Council, replaced the Dental Board referred to on page 28. The new body has nineteen members – five persons appointed by teaching bodies, seven registered dentists elected by the profession, two persons appointed by the Medical Council, one person appointed by the Minister for Education and four appointed by the Minister for Health, at least two of these being non-dentists representing consumer interests. The members have a term of office of five years and no member can hold office for more than two consecutive terms. The council is funded mainly by registration and retention fees. The Dental Council's functions vis-a-vis dentists and dentistry are similar to those of the Medical Council relating to medical practitioners. There is, however, no 'intern year' or provisional registration in the case of dentists.

Ordinarily, the practice of dentistry is confined by law to registered dentists (and doctors) but exceptions may be made, under conditions, for auxiliary dental workers and for students.[8] The Dental Council is considering the provisions which might be made for this.

There are two undergraduate training schools for dentists. One is managed in association with Trinity College by the Dublin Dental Hospital Board. It is planned that its activities will be transferred to a new dental school at St James's Hospital. The other school is in Cork in the grounds of the regional hospital at Wilton. It is run by University College, Cork. Qualifications in dentistry are conferred by the National University of Ireland (for Cork graduates), the University of Dublin and the Royal College of Surgeons (which is involved in postgraduate training). There are mutual provisions, like those for doctors, for recognition of qualifications of EC member states[9] and persons qualified in dentistry in non-EC countries may be registered where the Dental Board is satisfied as to the standard of qualification.[10]

In 1984, the number of dentists in Ireland was 1,131 (922 male and 209 female), 329 of these were employed wholetime by the health boards. Nearly all of the others were engaged in private practice and some 700 of them were involved in the scheme of dental benefits of the Department of Social Welfare.[11]

Nurses

The statutory controlling body for the nursing profession is an Bord Altranais (the Nursing Board). The present board was set up by the Nurses Act, 1985. It has twenty-nine members, categorised in an intricate pattern. Seventeen of the members are elected by the profession and the other twelve are appointed by the Minister for Health (at least three of the latter group must be doctors, others are representative of management and education and two are 'representative of the interest of the general public'). The term of office of members is five years. The board is financed mainly by examination, registration and retention fees payable by nurses.

160

The main functions of the board relate to:

1. the maintenance of a register of nurses, divided into categories as described below;
2. undergraduate training and examinations (the board itself does not provide undergraduate training but maintains a close control on it: it does conduct examinations itself);
3. postgraduate training, which it provides itself in some instances (in particular for public health nursing);
4. professional misconduct and fitness to practice;
5. the operation of EC directives relating to nursing.[12]

The board has, in relation to the training of nurses and midwives, powers more direct and detailed than those which the Medical Council has for doctors. The detailed syllabus for training is laid down by the board and the training hospitals must be approved by the board and must comply with its conditions for recognition. These conditions include provisions as to the size of the hospital, the teaching staff and the accommodation and facilities available to the student nurses.

The period of training for general, psychiatric and mental handicap nursing is three years and for the midwives division of the register one year. The combined periods are contracted in the case of a nurse studying for registration in a second division of the register.

Registration as a nurse entitles one to use the title of registered nurse and it is an offence for anyone who is not registered to use that title or to give the impression that she or he is registered. There is, however, no prohibition on anyone practising nursing. This is not so in midwifery. Attendance on women in childbirth is restricted by law, except where urgency makes this impracticable, to registered midwives and medical practitioners (and to bona fide students). Midwives practising their profession are supervised in their work by the health boards.[13]

Under the 1985 act, a new 'live' register of nurses has

been set up. On 1 January 1988, there were 28,000 names on this. The register is as yet incomplete. In 1986 there were 27 training schools for general nurses, four for sick children's nurses, seven for midwifery, nine for psychiatric nurses and six for mental handicap nurses. Since then, the number of training schools has been considerably reduced because of hospital closures and for other reasons. For example, the number taking in trainees for general nursing has been reduced to 13.[14]

Pharmaceutical chemists
The Council of the Pharmaceutical Society, a governing body of twenty-one for the pharmaceutical chemists of Ireland, was set up under the Pharmacy (Ireland) Act, 1975. The council is elected by the members of the society. Anyone who qualifies as a pharmaceutical chemist is entitled to be a member of the society as long as he continues to pay the annual fees required. Those who do not pay the annual membership subscriptions are licentiates of the society. They pay annual fees at a lower rate and have the same rights as members in the practice of pharmacy but have no say in the election of the council. One third of the members of the council go out of office each year. Registration fees, membership subscriptions and fees from students for the society's courses finance its activities.

The training of pharmaceutical chemists is a combination of an academic course of instruction with practical experience. A student wishing to become a pharmaceutical chemist must complete a four-year course of studies organised in the School of Pharmacy which is incorporated in the University of Dublin (Trinity College). This leads to the degree of Bachelor of Science (Pharmacy). Following this, there is a pre-registration year of practical experience under a tutor pharmacist at a place or places approved by the Pharmaceutical Society of Ireland. The student is then eligible for registration as a pharmaceutical chemist. About 50 graduate each year. There is a two-year diploma course for pharmaceutical technicians. This is provided partly by

Trinity College and partly by the Pharmaceutical Society.

Only those registered by the Pharmaceutical Society are permitted to 'keep open shop for retailing, dispensing or compounding poisons..... or medical preparations'. Pharmaceutical chemists also have a special status and responsiblities in dealing in dangerous narcotic drugs and certain other drugs which may be sold only on a medical or similar prescription.

There were 2,079 pharmaceutical chemists on the register on 1 October 1987. In addition, there were 738 assistants, 19 registered druggists and 14 dispensing chemists and druggists (a category with practically all the rights but not the title of pharmaceutical chemist). At that time there were 1,155 community pharmacies in the country, nearly all of which were in the general medical service referred to in chapter seven.[15] A study carried out in 1984 indicated that, of pharmacists in employment, 85% were in community pharmacy, 8% in hospital pharmacy and 4% in industry, the remainder being in wholesale trade and in academic and administrative posts.[16]

That study contains the following table showing the numbers of persons per community pharmacy in each EC country in January, 1982:

Table 2: *Persons per community pharmacy in the EC* (10)

Belgium	1,948
Denmark	16,352
Germany	4,035
France	2,829
Greece	2,209
Ireland	**2,872**
Italy	4,000
Luxembourg	5,352
Netherlands	13,333
United Kingdom	5,278

These figures reflect the differing arrangements for organising community pharmacy. Those countries with a high number of persons per pharmacy have large pharmacies employing a number of pharmacists.

Under EC directives and regulations made by the minister under the European Communities Act, 1972, qualifications obtained within the community by nationals of member states are recognised for registration as pharmaceutical chemist by the Pharmaceutical Society of Ireland. Irish nationals have similar rights in the other EC countries.[17]

Opticians
Bord na Radharcmhastoiri (The Opticians Board), set up under the Opticians Act, 1956, arranges for registration of opticians and supervises them in the practice of their profession. The board has eleven members made up of four registered medical practitioners, six opticians and one other person. The term of office of board members is five years. Its expenses are met from examination and registration fees and fees for courses of instruction given by it.

The board maintains two registers, one for ophthalmic opticians (who both prescribe and supply spectacles) and one for dispensing opticians (who supply spectacles only on the prescription of others). Those who undergo the courses of training and who pass the examinations prescribed by the board are registered. The board may also register foreign-trained opticians.

The board may itself provide training or may approve of other bodies to train opticians. Similarly, it may conduct the examinations or may appoint other bodies to do so under its rules. Post-registration courses for opticians may be provided. A four-year training course is arranged in the College of Technology, Kevin Street, Dublin.

The prescription of spectacles is confined to registered medical practitioners and ophthalmic opticians and dispensing of prescriptions is limited to these and to dispensing opticians. The sale of spectacles by unqualified persons is prohibited. Opticians, for their part, are restricted by law in their practice to the provision of spectacles and, in the case of ophthalmic opticians, their prescription. Opticians are specifically prohibited from treating eye disease, or from prescribing or administering drugs for that purpose or to paralyse the accommodation of the eye, and from suggesting that they are capable of making a medical diagnosis of eye disease. The board has made rules to regulate and control opticians in their practice and to control advertising by opticians. The titles of ophthalmic optician and dispensing optician are protected by the act.[18] On 1 January 1988, there were 298 registered ophthalmic opticians and 169 registered dispensing opticians. Not all of these are in wholetime practice as opticians.[19]

Other health professions

The above descriptions relate to those health professions for which there is statutory registration and control. Other professionals also make important contributions in the services. The major categories of these are described, in alphabetical order, in the following paragraphs.[20]

Chiropodists: About eighty chiropodists are employed in the public service. There is no recognised training school in the State (those employed here are trained in Belfast or in Britain, where there are three-year training courses).

Dieticians: There are about fifty dieticians in the public service. Training is provided at the College of Technology, Kevin Street, Dublin, which runs a four-year course leading to a diploma in dietetics and nutrition. There is a link with Trinity College, whereby students may obtain a university qualification.

Health inspectors: There are about 200 health inspectors in the public service. Their duties relate to food hygiene and other preventive health services and to environmental controls. There is a four-year training course in the College of Catering, Cathal Brugha Street, Dublin, which takes in about thirty students each year.

Medical laboratory technicians: There are about 850 medical laboratory technicians employed in the public service, as well as other specialised technicians, such as EEG/ECG technicians, of whom there are about fifty. There are training courses of three years' duration in the College of Technology, Kevin Street, the Cork Regional Technical College and the Galway Regional Technical College. The annual intake of students has been about forty-five.

Occupational therapists: There are about 130 occupational therapists in the public service. Training is provided in St Joseph's College, Dun Laoghaire under the control of the National Rehabilitation Board. The course lasts three years and the average annual intake of students is twenty-six.

Physiotherapists: There are about 400 physiotherapists in the public service. There are schools of physiotherapy in the Mater Hospital, Dublin and St James' Hospital, Dublin, each of which has an annual intake of about twenty-four. The schools are respectively associated with University College, Dublin and Trinity College, Dublin which grant diplomas.

Radiographers: There are about 500 radiographers in the public service. There are two training schools, both in Dublin – the School of Diagnostic Radiography, St Vincent's Hospital, and the School of Therapeutic Radiography, St Luke's Hospital, Dublin. The annual intake in St Vincent's is twelve and St Luke's takes in eight students in every second year – a total average annual intake of sixteen. This does not meet the full needs of the services and many of those in the service have been trained abroad. The recognised qualification for employment is the certificate of proficiency in radiography of the British-based Society of Radiographers.

Social workers: About 500 social workers are employed in the health services. The primary aim of social work is to help individuals, families and groups to deal with problems of living. Social workers are employed both in general medical care and in psychiatry. Courses leading to qualifications in social work are provided in University College, Dublin, Trinity College, Dublin and University College, Cork.

EMPLOYMENT IN HEALTH BOARDS.

Those in the health professions who are in entirely private practice are a small proportion of the total. Most work within the public system (largely the health boards and public

166

voluntary hospitals) either whole-time or in a combination of public and private practice. Most are salaried but in a few categories they are engaged on a contract basis, such as the

Figure 2: *Occupation*

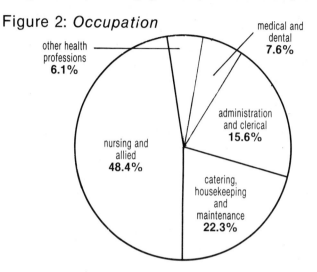

Figure 3: *Employing or contracting authority*

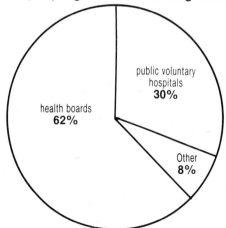

Note: 'Other' includes the Department of Health, the mental handicap homes and the central executive bodies described on page 148.

doctors and pharmacists in the general medical service. The total number of persons working in the public system, including those in the professions and others is about 58,000 (1984 figure) divided into the categories shown in Figures 2, 3, and 4.[21]

Figure 4: *Healthcare Programmes*

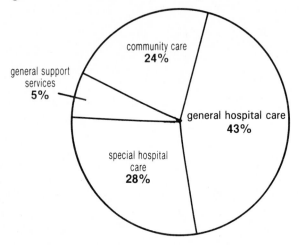

Note: 'Special hospital care' covers psychiatry, mental handicap, physical handicap, long-stay care, etc; 'community care' covers the general medical services, home nursing, dental, ophthalmic and aural services and the preventive and welfare programmes.

Personnel policy

The importance of an effective personnel policy to ensure the satisfactory functioning of the health services is widely recognised. This has been reflected both at health board and national level. At health board level there is a separate personnel function for each board, while in the structuring of the Department of Health special attention has been paid to the personnel function. The other health agencies, such as the voluntary hospitals and other voluntary organisations, also play a vital role both in the management of their own personnel and in the formulation of national policies for the various grades and types of staff.

The task confronting those involved in personnel issues in the health services is formidable in view of the number and variety of grades. These issues come under the following headings:

numbers, grades and recruitment

staff training and development

remuneration and conditions of service

formulation, implementation and monitoring of personnel policies in relation to specific related staff groups

liaison with the EC in directives for mutual recognition of qualifications, etc.

Numbers, grades and recruitment
Chapter II of Part II of the Health Act, 1970 provides a code governing the appointment and employment of personnel in health boards. The determination of the number and kinds of officers and servants to be appointed is made by the board in accordance with the directions of the minister. The making of appointments, and the determination of remuneration and conditions of employment are, however, reserved to the chief executive officer of the board and he, in taking decisions on these, must act in accordance with the directions of the minister. These directions are quite detailed and, with a summary of the legal provisions, are set out in Appendix G.

For the more senior classes of officer (including many of the professional posts) selection is made through the Local Appointments Commission. In other cases selection is made by the chief executive officer in accordance with a selection procedure specified by the minister. Qualifications for the various classes of officer under the health boards are determined by the minister. There is an age limit, normally sixty-five years, for employment.

The voluntary hospitals and other agencies are responsible

for the selection of their own staff. However, qualifications for those appointed and conditions of employment are substantially the same for similar grades of personnel whether employed by health boards or other health agencies.

Like those in other employments, health staff have benefited from many reforms which have taken place in the employment field in the recent past. Of these, the removal of the marriage bar in the public service and the Employment Equality Act, 1977 were particularly significant for the health services.

In the case of consultant medical staff, Comhairle na nOspideal plays an important role. It regulates the numbers and types of consultant appointments in hospitals providing services under the Health Acts and specifies professional qualifications for appointments.

Remuneration and conditions of service
Nearly all categories of health boards staffs are covered by a conciliation and arbitration scheme for health boards and local authorities. There is a national body – the Local Government Staff Negotiations Board[22] to represent management in the operation of this scheme. The Department of Health and the chief executive officers of the health boards are represented on it. Responsibility for the overall operation of the scheme is vested in a national joint council which consists of an equal number of members of the board and of the 'staff panel' (comprised of appropriate staff associations), under the chairmanship of an officer of the Labour Court. Some health board staff (notably psychiatric nurses and the non-officer grades) have access to the Labour Court. All staff employed by voluntary hospitals and other health bodies have access to the court. Permanent staff of health boards have the same superannuation scheme as those in local authorities.[23] It is a contributory scheme and provides for lump sum payments and pensions on retirement. There is also a contributory widows and orphans pension scheme for male staff. Salaried staffs in voluntary hospitals have similar arrangements for superannuation.

The consultants' contract

Prior to 1980, consultants in health board hospitals were paid by salary and those in the public voluntary hospitals by fees related to the number of days beds were occupied by their patients (an arrangement not conducive to efficiency in the throughput of patients). A working party representative of the department, Comhairle na nOspideal, the health boards, the voluntary hospitals and the professional organisations reported in 1978 recommending that these arrangements be replaced by a common form of contract for all public hospitals.[24]

This report described a consultant as follows:

A consultant is a registered medical practitioner in hospital practice who, by reason of his training, skill and experience in a designated specialty, is consulted by other registered medical practitioners and undertakes full clinical responsibility for patients in his care without supervision in professional matters by any other person. He will be a person of considerable professional capacity and personal integrity.

The working party recommended a new form of contract intended for application to all public hospitals. Its main features were:

— the model contract should be based on a commitment to public patients of twenty-seven hours of hospital sessions in a week (but individual contracts could be based on a smaller or greater number of hours),

— outside these sessions, a consultant could be rostered for availability for immediate attendance,

— attendances at the hospital for emergency duties outside ordinary hours would be covered,

— consultant appointments would be on a permanent basis,

— consultants would continue to be pensionable under the

Local Government (Superannuation) Act, 1956 or the
Voluntary Hospitals Superannuation Scheme,

— there would be an age limit of sixty-five years for all
consultant appointments,

— a consultant would be entitled to provision for private
practice at the hospital but the hospital authority could
limit the availability of this provision in certain
circumstances,

— private practice outside the hospital insofar as it did not
prevent the fulfilment of the terms of the contract would
not be restricted,

— the contract should be the subject of a complete general
review within a period of five years.

The remuneration of consultants under the contract has three
elements – payment for his scheduled commitments and for
any work arising within two hours of the end of that
commitment each day, payment for rostering outside these
hours and payment for individual attendances at the hospital
for emergencies arising outside these hours.

This contract has been in operation in most hospitals for
about seven years. A review of it has been announced by the
minister. This is particularly desirable in the light of the rise
in the numbers entitled to private care under the voluntary
health insurance schemes (see chapter sixteen).

This working party was also to report on a common
selection procedure for consultants.[25] There has been no
concrete development on this.

Continuing training
Health boards and voluntary hospitals have over the years
made an increased investment in terms of money, time and
effort in staff development. They are involved in the basic
training of many health professions.

Most of the money spent by health agencies on specialised
training is devoted to postgraduate training schemes provided

by the faculties of the medical schools, clinical societies, medical associations, university departments and to some extent private bodies. In addition, staff undergoing examinations for higher degrees or diplomas are granted special leave with pay and, in the case of whole-time medical, dental and nursing staffs, a fortnight's study leave with pay prior to the examination. An Bord Altranais provides post-qualification training for nurses and co-ordinates the activities of other bodies engaged in training for nurses.

Induction training is normally provided for administrative and clerical staffs by the employing health agency. Health agencies usually avail themselves of the courses provided by outside training and educational institutions to enable their staffs to acquire further interpersonal and management skills. In this area, the Institute of Public Administration is the largest training agency. It offers a degree course in public administration with a special option in health administration which is recognised by the National Council for Educational Awards. Courses are also run by the Institute of Hospital and Health Service Administrators, and the Irish Management Institute.

NOTES ON CHAPTER FOURTEEN

1. Under EC Directives 75/363 and 81/1057
2. Under section 27(2)(d) of the Medical Practitioners Act, 1978.
3. Section 29 of the 1978 act.
4. Section 59 of the 1978 act.
5. Source: unpublished study by the author, 1984
6. Source: Health Statistics, 1986 (Department of Health) and the above study
7. Source: Table H3, Health Statistics, 1986
8. Section 51 of the Dentists Act, 1985
9. Under EC Directives 78/686 and 81/1057
10. Section 27 of the 1985 act.
11. Source: Tables H2 and H9, Health Statistics, 1986 and Department of Social Welfare
12. The current directives are 77/452 and 81/1057
13. Under section 57 of the Nurses Act, 1985
14. Source: An Bord Altranais

15. Source: Pharmaceutical Society of Ireland and Table H8, Health Statistics, 1986
16. Corrigan O.I., CM Fisher and MC Henman, *Pharmacy Manpower in Ireland, 1983: Present Trends and Future Prospects*, School of Pharmacy, Trinity College, Dublin
17. Under EC Directives 85/432 and 85/433 and the European Communities (Recognition of Qualifications in Pharmacy) Regulations, 1987 (S.I. No 239 of 1987)
18. Sections 47 to 53 of the 1956 act
19. Source: Bord na Radharcmhastoiri
20. Source: unpublished study by the author, 1984.
21. The source for Figures 2–4 is mainly Table H1, Health Statistics, 1986
22. This body was set up by the Minister for the Environment under the Local Government (Corporate Bodies) Act, 1971
23. The Local Government (Superannuation) Act, 1956 was applied to health boards by section 20 of the Health Act, 1970
24. Working Party on a Common Contract and Common Selection Procedure for Consultants: Interim Report, 1978
25. Such a procedure was envisaged in section 41(1)(b)(v) of the Health Act, 1970

CHAPTER FIFTEEN

Finance

Customarily health expenditure is divided into non-capital and capital categories. These categories are not water-tight as expenditure on repairs and replacements met from current revenue is not always easily distinguishable from purely capital expenditure. With these reservations, the two types of expenditure are dealt with separately in this chapter.

NON-CAPITAL EXPENDITURE

Sources of non-capital expenditure
We have seen in earlier chapters how the basis for meeting the cost of the health services changed from local taxation, with a minor fraction of the cost met by central grants, to central taxation supplemented by local taxation. The share met by local taxation decreased, particularly after the health boards became responsible for the services in April, 1971 and ultimately, in the years 1973-76, the contribution from local taxation was phased out entirely. With the local rates no longer meeting any part of the cost, the sources of public finance in Ireland for the health services are now the Exchequer, health contributions from eligible persons and charges on persons using the services, which were introduced in 1987. An external source of finance was introduced upon entry into the EC under regulations governing member states' liability for the cost of health care for insured workers and pensioners. The hospitals sweepstakes, whose contribution to the running costs had diminished to 0.2% of the total by 1985, were wound up in 1986.

175

The percentages of expenditure met from each of these sources in the financial years to 31 March 1974 and 31 December 1985 were:

Table 1:[1]	*1973-4*	*1985*
	%	%
Exchequer	80.5	91.4
Rates	13.9	nil
Health contributions and some other items	3.8	6.6
Receipts under EC regulations	1.2	1.8
Hospital sweepstakes	0.6	0.2

Distribution of non-capital health funds to different agencies
The exchequer funds are voted each year and the amount is shown in the volume of estimates. The income from health contributions and from the EC is shown as an appropriation-in-aid to the health vote in that volume. In effect, this means that income becomes available, with the exchequer contribution, for distribution, by the Minister for Health to the health boards and other agencies. The volume of estimates shows, in the health vote, the broad headings for which the funds are to be used, and the classes of agencies to which the funds are distributed.

Health board finances
The health boards are, of course, the major agencies providing the services (indeed, the grants paid to most of the other agencies by the department are for services provided by them 'on behalf of health boards'). Therefore, the financial relationships between the minister and the health boards are the most significant of the financial arrangements for the services. These relationships are governed by Chapter III of Part II of the Health Act, 1970. The minister prescribes a standard form of accounts for health boards, appoints local government auditors to examine the accounts of the boards and submits the abstracts of accounts to the houses of the Oireachtas. Health boards are required to submit estimates

of receipts and expenditure to the minister in a form laid down by him. A health board is not permitted to incur expenditure for any service or purpose beyond the sum fixed for a particular period by the minister, and the chief executive officer of a board is charged with responsibility for seeing that this restriction is observed.

Distribution of non-capital expenditure by programmes
Health activities are grouped into programmes and, within each programme, services. The programmes and the services, with the expenditure for 1985, are itemised in Part 1 of Appendix H

The percentages of the gross expenditure on the different programmes in 1977 and in 1985 are shown in Figure 1.[2]

Figure 1: *Gross expenditure* %

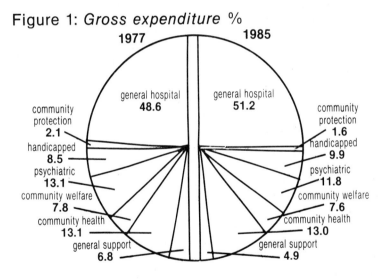

Distribution by the nature of items of expenditure
Figures 2, 3 and 4 below illustrate the allocation of expenditure for 1985 between public service pay and 'non-pay' items and, within each of these broad categories, the sub-division of items[3]:

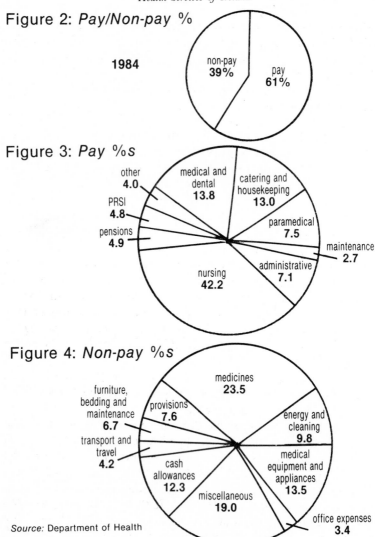

Figure 2: *Pay/Non-pay* %

1984

non-pay
39%
pay
61%

Figure 3: *Pay* %s

other
4.0
medical and
dental
13.8
catering and
housekeeping
13.0
PRSI
4.8
paramedical
7.5
pensions
4.9
maintenance
2.7
nursing
42.2
administrative
7.1

Figure 4: *Non-pay* %s

medicines
23.5
furniture,
bedding and
maintenance
6.7
provisions
7.6
energy and
cleaning
9.8
transport and
travel
4.2
medical
equipment and
appliances
13.5
cash
allowances
12.3
miscellaneous
19.0
office expenses
3.4

Source: Department of Health

Trends over the years in non-capital health expenditure
The trend in expenditure has been consistently upwards since
1947, in line with the extensions in the scope of the services
and the development of hospitals and other new facilities
described in earlier chapters. The cost in the year to 31

March, 1948 of the services then administered by local authorities was £5.7 million. It rose to £17.7 million by the year to 31 March, 1961 and to £61.5 million by the year to 31 March, 1971.

Much of these increases was due to the fall in the value of money over these years but, at constant money values, the rise was still substantial – from £5.7 million to about £15 million by the year ending March, 1961 and £33 million by the year ending March, 1971, when the health boards took over responsibility for the services. As percentages of gross national product, these figures also show a consistent rise. The percentage in 1947-48 was 1.7, in 1960-61 it was 2.6 and in 1970-71 it was 3.7.

The figures given above do not cover the totality of non-capital public expenditure on health care, only the part of it spent by the local authorities. Exchequer funds were also channelled elsewhere at this time by the Department of Health – in particular through the Hospitals Commission to the voluntary hospitals and other bodies. The figures cannot therefore be linked to those in the succeeding paragraphs, which relate to total public health expenditure in the years from 1971 on.

In the early nineteen-seventies, a number of new factors affected the trend in public health expenditure. First, there were the specific changes and improvements outlined in the 1966 white paper on the health services. These and the general expansionist drive pursued following the white paper ensured a continuance of the rise in expenditure noted in the preceding decades. There were other considerations which became more significant later in the nineteen-seventies. There was a rise in population (from 2,978,000 in 1971 to 3,443,000 in 1981, an increase of nearly 16 per cent). There were economic and financial disturbances, triggered by the crisis in oil prices following 1973, which included high rates of inflation. Generally, there was a liberal attitude in pay policy, in many cases leading to the concession of claims well in excess of the rate of inflation. Finally, for much of the decade, job creation in the public sector was specifically encouraged.

With this background, it is not surprising that health costs rose at an increased rate in the ninteen-seventies. At current prices, expenditure rose from £87 million in 1971-2 to £701 million in 1980. A more realistic comparison – at constant 1971 prices – shows an increase from £87 million to £212 million. Perhaps the most significant figures, however, are those for the cost per head of population, having regard to the substantial population rise. The cost per head of population in 1971-2 was £29.1 and in 1980 was £206.1 or, at constant 1971 costs, £62.3. Over the same period, the percentage of gross national product spent on the public health services and the ancillary welfare services under the Department of Health rose from 4.4 to 7.8.

The present decade has seen a change in the attitudes of successive governments towards public expenditure generally. This is shown in the figures for health expenditure. While the cost since 1980 rose in cash terms from £701 million to £1,169 million in 1985, at constant prices it fell from £212 million to £198 million and expenditure per head of population (at constant prices) fell from £62 to £56. The percentage of gross national product spent on the health and allied welfare services dropped from 7.8 to 7.5.

The table in Part 2 of Appendix H gives figures on the lines mentioned in the preceding paragraphs for each year

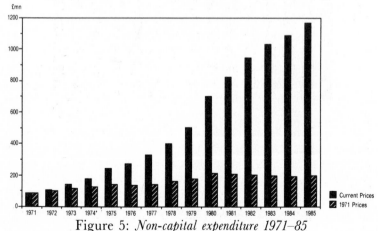

Figure 5: *Non-capital expenditure 1971–85*

from 1971-2 to 1985. Figures 5, 6 and 7 illustrate the trends.

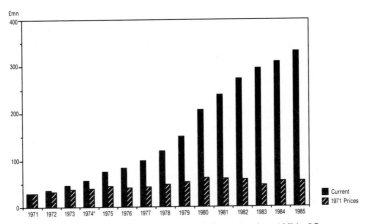

Figure 6: *Non-capital expenditure per capita 1971–85*

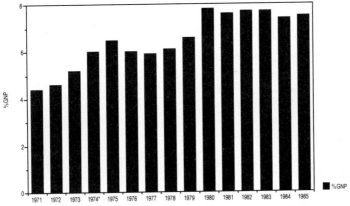

Figure 7: *Non-capital expenditure as a % of GNP*

International comparisons of health expenditure
It is difficult to compare the health expenditures of different
countries because of problems of definition, but there have
been a number of international studies in this field. In 1967,

Professor Brian Abel-Smith conducted a study for the World Health Organisation which compared health expenditure in thirteen varied countries. The percentage of gross national product shown in Professor Abel-Smith's study varied from 2.6 in the case of Finland to 4.3 in the case of Israel. The study related only to public expenditure and hence countries with a large private sector in the health field, such as the United States, showed a lower percentage of gross national product. Ireland was not a participant in this study but a calculation made in the Department of Health at the time showed that it would have been about half-way in the 'league-table' as represented by the proportion of gross national product.

A significant trend was mentioned in Professor Abel-Smith's study. This was that in high-income countries the proportion of gross national product spent on public health services generally rose at a rate equivalent to one per cent or more of gross national product every ten years. This was, indeed, the experience of Ireland during the nineteen-sixties.

More recently, the Organisation for Economic Co-operation and Development (OECD) published the results of a study which shows for each of its member states the percentages of gross domestic product (GDP) in that period which related to total health expenditure and to public health expenditure[4]. The study shows that, for twenty-three of the twenty-four members of OECD (Turkey's statistics were incomplete), both for total health expenditure and for public expenditure on health, there was a steady trend upwards. The average percentage of GDP for total health expenditure by OECD members rose from 4.1 in 1960 to 7.6 in 1983 and for public expenditure on health, the average percentage rose from 2.5 to 5.8. The highest percentage for public expenditure in 1983 was Sweden's, at 8.8. The highest for total health expenditure was the United States', at 10.8.

In using this study to compare Ireland's rate of spending on health care with other OECD countries, it is important to take account of the following reservation which was made in it on the calculation of our health costs:

The details shown suggest that Ireland has adopted a more comprehensive view of health than the sectoring recommended by SNA/COFOG and Eurostat; a reclassification of part of community welfare programmes and some other programmes would lower the ratio of GDP by up to one seventh in 1980.[5]

CAPITAL EXPENDITURE

The total amount of capital expenditure on the health services from public funds in any year is determined by the allocation given for this purpose in the health vote. The funds available are allotted by the Minister for Health to different agencies and for different purposes. Specific allocations of capital resources are decided on by the minister. In making his decisions he takes into account the national priorities for different categories of services and the needs of particular areas and particular institutions. In particular, where health board hospitals are concerned in capital development, the views of the health board in relation to priorities are given weight. The Department of Health supervises the spending of allocated moneys. Depending on the scale of expenditure and the type of project, this can vary from involvement in detailed specifications and plans to a general overall specification for accommodation and limits of cost.

In 1985, the capital allocation was £57 million, 45% of which was for health board projects and 55% for voluntary bodies. The allocation was divided among programmes as follows[6]:

Table 2: *Capital allocation 1985*

	£000
community health services (health centres etc)	1,379
community welfare services (welfare homes, etc)	1,195
psychiatric services	6,277
services for the handicapped	5,507
general hospital services	42,642

HEALTH CONTRIBUTIONS

Flat-rate contributions
The Health Contributions Act, 1971 introduced a new source of finance to meet part of the cost of the provision of services by health boards. This is a scheme of contributions by persons with limited eligibility towards the cost of the services available to them. The scheme of contributions was introduced on 1 October 1971, the rate of contribution then being 15 pence per week for insured workers and £7 a year for farmers, for other self-employed persons and for those with private means. At the same time, charges for hospital services formerly payable by those with limited eligibility were abolished. The rates for these contributions were increased periodically until they reached 50p per week and £24 a year in 1978.

Pay-related contributions
The 1971 act provided for the replacement of this scheme by one under which the contributions would be at a rate related to income and, in the case of farmers, generally to notional income based on valuation. This scheme commenced in April 1979.

The contributions under this new scheme were fixed at the rate of one per cent of income, up to a 'ceiling' of £5,500 a year. The contributions are collected with PRSI by the Revenue Commissioners.

Under this scheme, all income earners are liable to pay the health contributions, with the exception of persons with full eligibility and persons in receipt of certain social welfare benefits. Employers are liable to pay health contributions for employees with full eligibility.

The 'ceiling' for calculating contributions has been raised periodically. At present it is £15,000 a year. It will rise to £15,500 for the 1988-89 income tax year. The rate of contribution was raised from one per cent to one-and-a-quarter per cent in 1987.

184

COMMISSION ON HEALTH FINANCE

In 1987, the Minister for Health established a commission with the following remit:

To examine the financing of the health services and to make recommendations on the extent and sources of the future funding required to provide an equitable, comprehensive and cost-effective public health service and on any changes in administration which seem desirable for that purpose.

NOTES ON CHAPTER FIFTEEN

1. Source:1985 figures – table J2, Health Statistics, 1986; 1973–4 figures, Department of Health
2. Source:1977 figures, Department of Health; 1985 figures, table J1, Health Statistics, 1986
3. Source: Department of Health
4. *Measuring Health Care 1960-1983*, OECD, Paris 1985.
5. Ibid, page 23
6. Source: Health Statistics, 1986, table J5

CHAPTER SIXTEEN

Voluntary health insurance

Voluntary health insurance, as a means of providing for large numbers of the population, had been the subject of considerable discussion before the extended local authority services were decided upon in 1953. The new hospital and specialist services were designed to cater for the needs of some eighty-five per cent of the population. When these services had been introduced, there remained the issue of whether anything should be done to sponsor or encourage voluntary health insurance, particularly for those outside the 'health act' classes. The Minister for Health, Tom O'Higgins, appointed a special advisory body in January 1955 to examine this issue.

Report of advisory body
In their report to the minister in May 1956,[1] this advisory body found that voluntary health insurance benefits were provided on a very limited scale. The following is an extract from the relevant paragraph of the report:

> 7.... Few of the commercial insurance companies transact health insurance business and none does so to any material extent. One company introduced a scheme in 1953 offering hospital, medical and surgical benefits. It subsequently increased by 50 per cent the premium rates initially charged but, notwithstanding this, decided to terminate the scheme after about two years' experience. Some sickness benefits are provided through Friendly Societies of which about 100 are registered: of these some 30, with a total membership of approximately 17,000,

disburse sickness benefits in one form or another, and the total amount paid each year is about £17,000. In addition, there are a number of schemes associated with particular firms or organisations which provide sickness benefits for their members, generally in the form of contributions towards hospital and medical expenses.

In approaching their terms of reference, the advisory body assumed that the primary objective on which they were asked to advise was protection against the high and unforeseeable cost of ill-health and not against the minor costs which can readily be allowed for in the family budget. The benefits which the advisory body thought should be given under such a scheme were maintenance in hospital or nursing home, surgical and medical fees (in accordance with a graduated scale for major, intermediate and minor operations), maternity benefit, drugs and medicines for hospital in-patients, medical and surgical appliances, and various specialist services for in-patients in hospital. The body recommended that specialist medical services given outside hospitals and dental treatment should not be covered. They also thought that no benefit should be included for the supply of drugs and medicines, except for persons in hospital. The report recommended that in any scheme there should be a waiting period before acceptance of three months, except for claims arising from accidents, and that the insurance should be on the basis of annual contracts.

Having considered the possiblities of the operation of their suggested scheme by various types of agencies and having commented on the practice in other countries, the body advised:

> We are not aware that there are any interests in this country prepared to establish a health insurance scheme of the kind mentioned in our terms of reference and if a scheme is to be introduced, the State must take the initiative. A scheme could be administered by a Department of State, but we think it would have a wider

187

appeal to the public if it were administered by a company such as we describe.'

The company envisaged by the advisory body was one which would be guaranteed by the State, at least at its commencement, and which would not be obliged to comply with the provisions in the Insurance Acts relating to the licensing of insurance companies.

On the basis of the figures available to it, the body reached the general conclusion that, although a voluntary health insurance scheme would increase the income of voluntary hospitals, the increase was unlikely to be appreciable in relation either to the total income of those hospitals or to their annual deficits.

A calculation in the report of the advisory body shows that at the time it was prepared, there were some 457,000 persons not entitled to the health services under the Health Act, 1953 and thus potential clients for a voluntary health insurance scheme. The body thought that if persons eligible for health act services who might be disposed to become members were included, the total potential number of participants would be in the region of 500,000. They cautioned, however, that:

> one would have to assume that the number of persons who would be likely to join a scheme, particularly at its commencement, would be considerably less than the figure mentioned.

The recommendations of the advisory body were accepted, with some exceptions, and were the basis of the Voluntary Health Insurance Act, 1957.

The Voluntary Health Insurance Board
Under this act a new board, the Voluntary Health Insurance Board, was set up. The chairman and four other members are appointed by the minister and have a five-year term of office. The board is charged with providing health insurance

188

schemes. It is a non-profit-making body, any surplus on its income being devoted to the reduction of premiums or increase in benefits.

The board's schemes

When the board commenced business in October, 1957, it offered three separate schemes. The basic scheme provided for maintenance benefit at the rate of £6 6s a week, with further benefits to cover medical and surgical fees and other expenses in hospitals. Two other schemes were introduced at the same time, giving higher benefits of the same type for higher premiums. There was no provision in any of these schemes for normal maternity care.

After some years' operation of the schemes, the board changed over to more flexible provisions, whereby the policy-holders could choose the cover which they wished to take out for maintenance or treatment. However, its new schemes, introduced in April 1979, reverted to the concept of three general plans. These were designed to complement the changes in eligibility for the public services which were made at that time.

At the time of writing the board has five basic plans:

Plan A, giving full cover for semi-private accommodation in public hospitals and partial cover for private accommodation in those hospitals and for care in private hospitals,

Plan B, covering private or semi-private accommodation in public hospitals and semi-private accommodation in private hospitals, excluding the Blackrock Clinic and the Mater Private Hospital, and partially covering care in the latter institutions and care in private rooms generally.

Plan C, covering private and semi-private accommodation in all classes of hospitals, with the exception of the Blackrock Clinic and the Mater Private Hospital, and partially covering care in them,

Plan D, providing cover as in Plan C but also covering

fully semi-private accommodation in the Blackrock Clinic and The Mater Private Hospital and,

Plan E, covering private or semi-private accommodation in all hospitals, including the Blackrock Clinic and the Mater Private Hospital.

The premiums payable to the board are graded in relation to the cover given and the number of dependants covered. They include an element to cover professional fees at a level recommended by the board.

In addition to covering hospital costs, each plan includes an annual benefit for out-patient expenses. These include general practitioners' and consultants' fees, the cost of prescribed drugs (to the extent not met by the health boards' refund scheme, see page 87) home nursing and specified medical and surgical appliances. The first £170 in a year for a family or £105 for an individual is not covered and there are cash limits for each plan on the amount of the benefit.

A separate plan was introduced by the board in May, 1987, to allow for insurance against the liability to pay the hospital charges introduced at that time (see page 128). This is available to persons not participating in the board's other schemes.

The board has detailed rules on the operation of its schemes. They specify a number of limitations on benefits. Benefit for in-patient care is limited generally to 180 days in any subscription year and, in cases of alcoholism or drug or other substance abuse, benefit is restricted to a total aggregate period of 91 days (the rule in this case states, however, 'this benefit will be reinstated after five years' continuous membership since the last in-patient treatment, provided that the member has remained free of the condition during that period and has completed a course of aftercare recognised by the board').

There are general restrictions on the board's liability for medical conditions arising before a person is registered for insurance. No benefit will be payable for any such condition but this restriction will be removed after five years for persons who entered into membership under the age of fifty-five, after seven years for those who entered under sixty and after ten years for those who are aged sixty or over on entry. The upper age limit for entry is sixty-four years (until 1987 it was sixty-five). Except in some specific cases, benefits are not payable for conditions arising within a period after entry which ranges from thirteen to twenty-six weeks, depending on age at entry.[2]

The board's clientele
The numbers covered by the board's scheme have increased steadily since it commenced business. The growth in membership since 1978 is illustrated in Figure 1 below.[3]

Figure 1: *Membership growth 1978-87*

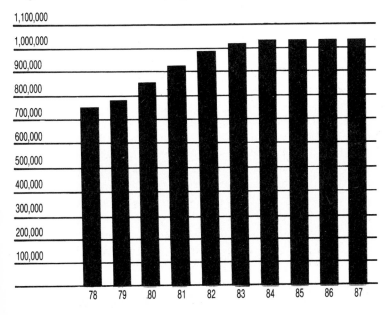

The board's finances
In the year to 28 February 1987 subscription income came to £112m. and claims totalled £110m. Administration expenses were £7m. and investment income came to £7m. At the end of the financial year, the board held £29m. in reserves. During the year 121,756 persons were assisted through payment of claims for in-patient hospital services and 26,005 claimed for day-care treatment at hospitals. £14.1m. was paid out to meet 66,399 claims for general practitioner and related services.[4]

Licensing of other insurers
By the Voluntary Health Insurance Act, 1957 health insurance was freed from the controls exercised on insurance businesses generally under the Insurance Acts, 1909 to 1953. Instead, it was made necessary for any person (with some exceptions – the most important being trade unions and friendly societies) wishing to provide health insurance to hold a licence from the Minister for Health. These licences are issued only for limited types of insurance schemes which are not seriously competitive with those of the Voluntary Health Insurance Board.

To provide health insurance without a licence (where such is required) or to pay a subscription or premium to a person doing this is an offence.[5]

Income tax relief on voluntary health premiums
Subscriptions for voluntary health insurance may be claimed in the succeeding year as deductions from income in the calculation of income tax. The full amount paid is deductible so that, at current rates of taxation, those liable for income tax at the standard rate obtain relief to the extent of about one-third of what they pay for voluntary health insurance. Those taxed at higher rates obtain more relief.

The Commission on Taxation in its first report in 1982[6] made the following comment and recommendation:

10.68 Relief is allowed for income tax purposes in respect of medical insurance premiums paid in the year preceding the year of assessment. This was introduced in 1955 to encourage the development of the Voluntary Health Insurance Board which had just been established (*sic*). While the Voluntary Health Insurance Board is the main body carrying on medical insurance, licences under the Voluntary Health Insurance Act, 1957 have been issued to a number of other bodies. Premiums payable to these bodies also qualify for relief.

10.69 Since the relief was introduced, the provision of public health services has been extended. In particular, hospital care in a public ward is now provided free of charge to all persons at the point of use. Heavy expenditure on drugs in the case of long-term illnesses is also reimbursed by health boards. Furthermore, the Voluntary Health Insurance Scheme has become well-established and widely used. Quite apart from the question of tax relief the value of such insurance is now appreciated widely. Accordingly, we recommend that the relief should now be abolished.

Income tax refunds for health expenses
Income tax payers may obtain some relief on heavy private expenditure on health care through a scheme operated by the Revenue Commissioners. If, in any year, the amount of expenditure for an individual which is not met from public funds or insurance is greater than £50, any excess qualifies for a special rebate of income tax. These limits apply to each dependant of the taxpayer individually and not to the total costs incurred by the taxpayer on himself and his dependants. A separate calculation is made for each. The scheme extends to most forms of medical and ancillary treatment but not to routine ophthalmic or dental treatment.

Claims under the scheme are made after the end of the tax year in question and the refund is calculated at the standard taxation rate. For example, if there has been expenditure of £160 on a taxpayer or a dependent, the taxpayer will get a refund of £38.50 (£160 less £50=£110, at 35p in the £=£38.50). The rebate only applies, of course, if that amount of tax, or more, has been paid. The scheme is thus a useful aid to those who pay income tax. The Commission on Taxation in its first report recommended some modifications in this scheme.

International Federation of Voluntary Health Service Funds
This international body has its headquarters in Ireland and is incorporated here under the International Health Bodies (Corporate Status) Act, 1971. The aims and purposes of the federation, which had its origins in a decision taken at the first International Conference on Voluntary Health Insurance held in Dublin in 1966, are to assist individuals in obtaining health services and for this purpose to promote the development and study of voluntary non-profit health services throughout the world.

Membership of the federation, which is a non-profit-making body, is open to organisations carrying out, or co-ordinating, voluntary health services on a non-profit basis, other organisations interested in voluntary non-profit health services, and persons interested in voluntary non-profit health services. The Voluntary Health Insurance Board is a member of the federation.

NOTES ON CHAPTER SIXTEEN

1. Report of Advisory Body on Voluntary Health Insurance Scheme (Prl 3571), 1956, Stationery Office, Dublin
2. The information on the board's schemes is based on its hospital directory (December 1987) and its rules (July 1987), obtainable from the Voluntary Health Insurance Board's offices
3. Report and Accounts, 1987, Voluntary Health Insurance Board.
4. Ibid.
5. The provisions on these matters are in sections 22 to 25 of the 1957 act
6. First Report of the Commission on Taxation, July, 1982 (Pl 617), page 148

CHAPTER SEVENTEEN

The future – a personal view

At the time of writing, the restrictions on the health services of the early nineteen-eighties are continuing and have been intensified. Lack of economic growth and fiscal problems arising from accumulated debt have led to the contribution to the health services from tax revenue being substantially reduced in real terms. In the absence of alternative sources of finance of significance, this means that expenditure on the services in real terms is falling. The figure on page 180 shows this for the period up to 1985 and it can be expected that the figures for 1986, 1987 and 1988 will show a deepening of this trend.

This seems inescapable in present circumstances (but, as is said below, a re-arrangement of Exchequer commitments in the health area generally could ease the position of the public health care system considerably). If the results achieved from the development of the health services are not to be seriously reversed, attention must centre in the first place on possible changes in the health care system to meet the altered circumstances and in the second place, on the financing of the system and possible changes in the financial arrangements.

THE HEALTH CARE SYSTEM

The public health care system originated with the concept of providing basic care for the poor and it progressed in the present century to the organisation of services for an increasing proportion of the population, in line with the rising cost of health care associated with the more sophisticated

195

techniques and facilities which became available. Thus the needs to be met by the services changed over time and the objectives of the system altered with the needs. The restructuring of the health services since the second world war described in this book and their augmentation from time to time followed a general trend in developed countries (in the twenty-four OECD countries, for example, the average percentage of GDP allocated to health care roughly doubled between 1960 and 1983).

Questions on the size and range of health care systems are being increasingly asked throughout the world. Are they too costly in relation to the results obtained? Are there better ways of meeting needs? Can more effective results be achieved in other ways (for example, by concentrating on care in the community rather than in institutions)? Can administration be bettered? These are among the questions being asked. They are not new in Ireland but they have a special impact now in view of our financial situation.

On the general issue of the scale of expenditure, there is no simple answer. There is no formula to indicate what is the right percentage of GNP or GDP which need be and should be represented by the cost of health care. In OECD countries, the percentages for total expenditure, public and private, for 1983 ranged from 4.7 for Greece to 10.8 for the United States and 9.6 per cent for Sweden. Ireland's percentage, as shown in the study, was about 8 per cent. For public expenditure alone, the highest published figure was 8.8 per cent for Sweden and the second highest was for Ireland at 7.5 per cent. However, because our view of the range of care covers elements of community welfare excluded by the other countries, the Irish figures should, to obtain a real comparison, be discounted by one-seventh (see page 183), putting them at about 6.9 per cent for total expenditure and 6.4 per cent for public expenditure on actual health care, the OECD averages for 1983 being 7.6 per cent and 5.8 per cent.[1]

One general trend can be seen in the OECD figures. The richer a country becomes, the higher is the proportion of its wealth which is devoted to health care. Estimates for 1986 show the United States spending over 11 per cent of GNP on health and West Germany over 9 per cent.[2] This trend seems to exist whether care is provided mainly through the public sector or through the private sector. Two points can be made from this. First, wealth does not ensure health and, secondly, there is no discerned limit to the proportion of its wealth which a country may reasonably devote to health care. For less rich countries, where the percentages are considerably lower, there are always unfilled needs in the field of health care. Hence, endeavours must lie in ensuring the efficiency of the system and in reducing the incidence of ill health.

Turning to the Irish system, the first question is: is it overblown and inefficient? The part of the system in which this question mostly arises is the general hospital service, the most expensive element in it.

In chapter eleven, the efforts, still uncompleted, towards rationalising the general hospital system have been described. However, even as it has been up to now, this system does not show up as being inefficient vis-a-vis other EC countries. The number of beds per 1,000 population, as recorded in 1976, was the second lowest in the community. Admission rates to general hospitals were similar to those for most EC countries and the throughput of patients per bed (28) was the highest in the EC (see pages 128–29). Furthermore, there has been no great change in the number of general hospital beds in Ireland since 1971, while the population has risen by about one fifth. While one may hold some reservations on whether all of those admitted to hospital need to be there, rather than being catered for in the community, one must conclude from these statistics that our system measured up well in the sense of dealing with the numbers seeking hospital care.

Similar considerations may arise in our psychiatric services but in this case, the ratio of hospital beds to population in Ireland in 1976 was 4.9 per 1,000, the highest in the EC[3]. As described in chapter nine, the policy for some time has been to cut down on hospital admissions for psychiatric care in favour of community care. This is reflected in the statistics shown in that chapter.

The principle of giving preference to community care cannot be contested. Throughout most of the periods discussed in earlier chapters there was proper emphasis on this – from the introduction of the dispensary system and the preventive services in the last century to more recent developments such as the expansion of the home nursing service, the introduction of the 'choice-of-doctor' scheme for the lower income group and of schemes to subsidise supplies of drugs and medicines for others. However, because of the expansion of medical knowledge and the development of new techniques and equipment that could only be applied and used in the organised environment of the hospital, resources were attracted increasingly to the general hospital system and the proportion of the health budget allocated to the hospital increased inexorably.

Currently there is a reaction to this, with pressure for the transfer to the community of part of the work done in the hospitals. This work ranges from simple care in district hospitals to sophisticated treatment in the major general and specialist hospitals. Much of the first kind of care could be carried out in the community if the services there were geared to it (indeed, the district hospitals, serviced as they are by general practitioners, can almost be regarded now as part of the community services). For the rest, there must be doubts as to how much could be done in the community as effectively as in hospitals. At present, it is thought that of those with ill-health who have contact with the health system, over ninety per cent are dealt with by community-based services. Of the remainder, who go to hospital, nearly all are filtered through community doctors who regard them as needing treatment at a hospital. It is questionable therefore whether there are large numbers of those admitted to hospital at present who could be treated suitably in the community.

In the long-term, a substantial reduction in the number receiving hospital care might be achieved by prevention of

the conditions which cause people to go to hospital. The five
conditions which account for sixty per cent of bed-days in
general hospitals (see page 127) are preventible to varying
degrees but prevention requires changes in life-style which
can only be achieved over time. Heart disease and other
diseases of the circulatory system are directly linked to diet
and life-style and the incidence of these diseases in Ireland is
exceptionally high. Other countries – notably Finland and
the United States – have achieved reductions in the incidence
of these diseases through educational programmes designed
to improve life-style and eating habits and Ireland can do
the same (the initiative of the Kilkenny Health Project is
described on page 81). Diseases of the respiratory system are
often linked to smoking. The controls on this habit are
outlined in chapter six. Accidents, poisoning and violence
could, perhaps, be reduced by further educational efforts.
The incidence of the fourth and fifth of these conditions,
diseases of the digestive system and neoplasms, can be
similarly reduced.

In the psychiatric programme, conditions associated with
alcohol abuse and drug dependance rank high in the reasons
for hospitalisation. Here again, public authorities have scope
to control the incidence, by educational programmes and
through fiscal arrangements and the regulation of the
availability of alcohol.

It should not be thought that emphasis on community
care and the adoption of better-informed life-styles will
quickly reduce pressure on the health care system, and on
the hospitals in particular. The kind of changes needed
involve dietary and other adjustments affecting many
industrial and commercial interests, including the manufacturers and distributers of foods, tobacco and alcoholic drinks,
and the producers of dairy products, meat and sugar and
will require departures from some traditional Irish habits.
Change may be slow and it is not possible to be confident
that pressure on the curative health services will be greatly
reduced in the short term or in the medium term.
Furthermore, developing technology, particularly in hospitals,

is likely to continue to offer opportunities to cure or alleviate some conditions not treatable in the past. Thirty years ago, few would have foreseen the technology which now exists for heart surgery, brain surgery, artificial joints and eye operations, to cite some examples.

FINANCE

Whatever changes the future may bring in the health care system, it is clear that the financing of the system must be closely examined (as it will be, no doubt, by the commission referred to on page 185). In 1983, it was estimated that over three-quarters of the total cost of health care in Ireland was met from public funds and it is not thought that the proportion has changed materially since. The Exchequer in 1985 met ninety-one per cent of the cost of public non-capital expenditure (the balance was met mainly by health contributions and receipts under EC regulations). Hence, if the Exchequer contribution is reduced in real terms, either the health system must be contracted or other sources of finance, public or private, must be found.

Other sources of finance
What other sources of public finance are possible? Local taxation may be ruled out. There is no replacement of the rates system now evident which would finance local authority contributions to the health services (such as were provided for in the 1970 Health Act)[4] and for local authorities to pay contributions which would be financed largely by the Exchequer grants now paid to them would solve nothing. Health contributions could contribute more if the rate was increased above the present level of $1\frac{1}{4}$ per cent but these now seem to be widely regarded as simply another form of taxation. Charges on patients for services, particularly in or at hospitals, provide some revenue but can be administratively cumbersome. Thinking in other fields is needed if there is to

be substantial relief to the Exchequer without excessive diminution of the services.

Lotteries are a possibility. While funds from the national lottery are allocated to health care, there could also be scope for local lotteries and other fund-raising activities for specific projects. These are common now in the case of the voluntary hospitals. Health boards could be encouraged to follow this example by stimulating local groups to raise money (section 33 of the 1970 act envisaged the health boards accepting gifts).

Another possibility could lie in extending to other classes of injury and illness the principle whereby the cost of treatment arising from road accidents is recoverable from the persons liable for causing the injury (see page 128). Examples might be injuries at work (where the cost could be made payable by the employer) and sports injuries (where organisers could be made liable). A further extension of this principle could allow for levies on industries producing, advertising and distributing products which were known to cause or contribute to conditions which impose demands on the health care system (the tobacco industry is an obvious example).

The Exchequer's role
In considering the Exchequer's role vis-a-vis the financing of the health care system, it is necessary to look beyond the health vote, which shows only the outgoings to meet expenditure by the health agencies, and to examine more broadly the relationship of health care to the revenue and outgoings of the Exchequer. In particular, attention should be given to the financing of voluntary health insurance. The income of the Voluntary Health Insurance Board comes mainly from subscriptions paid by its clients. These subscriptions are tax-deductible (see page 192). Subscriptions in the year to February 1987 totalled £110 million.[5] If, on average, there were deductions from members' income tax liability at the standard rate of thirty-five per cent (a conservative assumption) in respect of their subsriptions, the Exchequer lost almost forty million pounds.

In 1982, the Commission on Taxation recommended the ending of this concession (see page 192). Since then the case for this has become stronger. When the voluntary health insurance scheme was introduced in 1957, it was intended basically for the higher income group, the top fifteen per cent or so of the population, which was not eligible for general hospital care (except in a few special categories). Hence, the tax concession to encourage this group to partake in the insurance scheme. The scheme has grown to cover over a million people, about thirty per cent of the population. All of those covered are now eligible for public hospital care. As private hospitals have only about eight per cent of the general hospital beds in the country (1984 figure), it seems that most of the care for voluntary health insurance clients is given in public hospitals. In these hospitals, the only apparent advantages for those covered by voluntary health insurance is in having access to private and semi-private accommodation and in being private patients of the consultants. In the current condition of the national finances, it is surely extravagant for the state to subsidise by way of tax concession those who participate in voluntary health insurance to gain these advantages.

With regard to the Exchequer's role, another point should be borne in mind. Because of the high pay content in health expenditure, any sums allocated to the health agencies should, to show the net effect on the Exchequer, be discounted by the direct taxes deducted at source or otherwise paid by health personnel. If the tax concession for voluntary health insurance was ended and the sum saved was diverted to the health vote, thereby permitting some additions to personnel, considerably more than £40 million could be added to the money available for the health services, with a net effect on the Exchequer which would be neutral.

PAYING FOR HEALTH CARE IN THE FUTURE

Whatever might be done on the above lines or otherwise to

ease the present constraints on the Exchequer's contribution, the wants and needs of the future will call for some fundamental thinking on the ways to provide health care and specifically on the roles of the state and of private agencies.

For some of the programmes described in earlier chapters it would be difficult to justify any major change in the existing system of organisation and finance. These are the community protection programme, which is for the good of all, and the community welfare and handicap programmes. Public expenditure on these three programmes accounts for 19 per cent of non-capital expenditure on the services. Most would agree that this would apply also to the 'choice-of-doctor' scheme, which accounts for 9 per cent of the expenditure.

These services are mostly for categories of persons who would have little capacity to contribute from private resources to the cost but for the other programmes (particularly the general hospital and psychiatric programmes) eligibility is wider, generally extending to the whole population. Almost 70 per cent of the expenditure goes on these programmes. It is among them that changes to reduce the Exchequer liability in one way or another are likely to be fruitful. Within these programmes, all but a small fraction of the services are provided in public hospitals. The private hospitals and homes complement these. One issue is whether there should be a change in the ratio between the public and private sectors to relieve the former by encouraging the latter. The present policy of rationalising the public hospitals, which coincides with some new private initiatives, is changing this ratio, but not to a very significant extent. Hence, the financial problem seems essentially to relate to the cost of the public hospital system or, more accurately, to the extent to which the Exchequer can meet this cost.

It seems clear that, at least for a number of years, some way to supplement the Exchequer from other sources should be sought. The charges on patients introduced in 1987 are an example of this but, as flat-rate charges like these must be related to what a person with an income just above the 'medical card' limit can afford, the funding available from them is limited. More income could be raised if charges like these were related to incomes.

A broad approach on these lines could require that, right across this group of programmes, those using them, except for medical card holders, would have to pay the cost of the services required up to a specified limit, graded in relation to income. Public funds would only meet the cost in excess of this limit. For example, instead of the present charges, a user of the services could be required to pay up to a fixed percentage of monthly income for services provided in any month. Such an approach could have the incidental advantage of removing an existing anomaly whereby care in the community can be more costly to individuals than hospital care.

An alternative would be to reduce public expenditure by privatising part of the system, including the ownership of some of the present public institutions, and cutting down substantially on eligibility for the services. This is not an appealing option. The social implications are repellent and there is evidence that its outcome would be undesirable from an economic point of view. The United States, where about sixty per cent of health expenditure is in the private sector, has the highest figure for total health expenditure as a percentage of GDP and its health system does not seem to give satisfaction. The following comment is revealing:

> The rising cost of American health care is forcing patients to treat themselves. Those who are being discharged from hospitals quicker and sicker are becoming the customers of a fast-expanding industry that supplies the helpers and hardware needed for invalids to cope at home....... Patients in America will, for instance, this year spend around $1.1 billion on respirators for use in their homes, $350 million on dialysis machinery, $550 million on infusions and $190 million on wheelchairs.[6]

ADMINISTRATION

The question 'can administration be bettered' was posed earlier in this chapter. Betterment should certainly be sought and any administration should, after a period of years, be closely examined to see if it is what is best suited for current needs. However, I will conclude with the following advice from a well-known authority on organisation and administration:

> It must be considered that there is nothing more difficult to carry out, nor more doubtful of success nor more dangerous to handle, than to indicate a new order to things, for the reformer has enemies in all those who profit by the old order and only lukewarm defenders in all those who would profit by the new.[7]

NOTES TO CHAPTER SEVENTEEN

1. *Measuring Health Care 1960-1983*, OECD, Paris, 1985, page 12.
2. *The Economist*, 4 July, 1987, page 20.
3. Health Statistics, 1981, Table E8.
4. Section 32.
5. Voluntary Health Insurance Board, Report and Accounts, 1986.
6. *The Economist*, July 25, 1987, page 62.
7. Machiavelli, N, *The Prince*.

APPENDIX A

Full eligibility

PART 1
GUIDELINES FOR ELIGIBILITY, 1987

Income Limits   *£ per week*
single person living alone
  — under 66 years... 68.50
  — 66 to 80 years.. 73.50
  — over 80 years... 76.50

single person living with family
  — under 66 years... 56.50
  — 66 to 80 years.. 61.50
  — over 80 years... 64.50

married couple
  — under 66 years... 98.50
  — 66 to 80 years.. 108.50
  — over 80 years... 114.50

Allowances added to above figures
  — each child under 16 years............................... 11.00
  — each other dependent...................................... 12.50
  — outgoings on house *in excess of*...................... 11.00
  — expenses on travelling to work *in excess of*....... 9.50

PART 2

NUMBERS COVERED BY MEDICAL CARDS ON 1 OCTOBER
1987

Health board	Number of persons (including dependants) covered	Percentage of population covered
Eastern		
Dublin	302,941	29.68
Wicklow	35,269	37.33
Kildare	41,955	36.16
TOTAL	380,165	30.88
Midland		
Longford	15,067	47.85
Westmeath	24,496	38.69
Offaly	23,945	40.04
Laois	21,345	40.07
TOTAL	84,853	40.82
Mid-Western		
Clare	31,712	34.72
Limerick	54,995	33.49
Tipperary (NR)	21,457	36.09
TOTAL	108,164	33.34
North Eastern		
Cavan	24,458	45.39
Louth	44,938	49.01
Meath	40,752	39.27
Monaghan	22,793	43.55
TOTAL	132,941	44.07

North Western		
Donegal	73,055	56.44
Leitrim	13,325	49.35
Sligo	21,939	39.19
TOTAL	108,319	51.00
South Eastern		
Carlow	17,518	42.77
Kilkenny	30,110	41.19
Tipperary (SR)	37,173	48.24
Waterford	33,143	36.38
Wexford	40,171	39.21
TOTAL	158,115	41.11
Southern		
Cork	146,490	35.50
Kerry	51,823	41.82
TOTAL	198,313	36.96
Western		
Galway	76,811	43.11
Mayo	61,332	53.32
Roscommon	26,983	49.46
TOTAL	165,126	47.48
GRAND TOTAL	1,335,996	37.71

Source: General Medical Services (Payments) Board.

APPENDIX B

Notes on law on control of infectious diseases

These notes are a guide to the legal provisions operative on 1 January 1988 but anyone needing a precise detailed knowledge of them should refer to the legal texts and to any changes made hereafter in them.

The law on the control of infectious diseases is contained in Part IV of the Health Act, 1947 (No. 28 of 1947), (as amended by sections 34 to 37 of the Health Act, 1953 (No. 26 of 1953)), the second schedule to the 1947 act, the Infectious Diseases Regulations, 1981 (S.I. No. 390 of 1981)), as amended by the Infectious Diseases (Amendment) Regulations, 1985 (S.I. No. 268 of 1985)), the Infectious Diseases (Shipping) Regulations, 1948 (S.I. No 170 of 1948) and the Infectious Diseases (Aircraft) Regulations, 1948 (S.I. No 136 of 1948).

Specification of infectious diseases
Under section 29 of the 1947 act, the minister 'may by regulations specify the diseases which are infectious diseases'. The current specification, in article 6 and the schedule to the 1981 regulations (as amended by the 1985 regulations), is:

acute anterior poliomyelitis
acute encephalitis
acute viral meningitis
anthrax
bacillary dysentery
bacterial meningitis (including
    meningococcal   septicaemia)
brucellosis
cholera
diphtheria
food poisoning (bacterial other
    than salmonella)
gastro enteritis (when
    contracted by children
    under two years of age)
infective mononucleosis
influenzal pneumonia
legionnaires disease
leptospirosis
malaria
measles
ornithosis
plague
rabies
rubella
salmonellosis (other than typhoid
or paratyphoid)

sexually transmissible diseases
— syphilis
— gonorrhoea
— chancroid
— lymphorgranuloma
    venereum
— granuloma inguinale
— non-specific urethritis
— chlamydia trachomatis
— trachomoniasis
— candidiasis
— pediculosis pubis
— ano-genital warts
— molluscum contagiosum
— genital herpes simplex
smallpox
tetanus
tuberculosis
typhoid and paratyphoid
typhus
viral haemorrhagic diseases
    (including lassa fever and
    marburg disease)
viral hepatitis
— type A
— type B
— type unspecified
whooping cough
yellow fever

General duty to take precautions
A person who 'knows that he is a probable source of infection with an infectious disease' must, 'take every other reasonable precaution to prevent his infecting others with such disease by his presence or conduct or by means of any article with which he has been in contact'. Similar precautions must be taken as respects a person in one's care who is a probable source of infection (section 30 of the 1947 act).

Regulations

Section 31 of the 1947 act (as amended by section 34 of the 1953 act) specifies the minister's power to make regulations 'providing for the spread (including the spread outside the State) of an infectious disease or of infectious diseases generally and for the treatment of persons suffering therefrom'. The second schedule to the act lists a number of matters which may be covered by such regulations.

Exemption from compulsory immunisation, etc

Section 32 deals with exemptions from compulsory immunisation or other measures which may be prescribed by regulations under section 31. As the 1981 regulations make no provision for such compulsory measures, this section of the act is in abeyance.

Precautions relating to dwellings

Sections 33 to 36 of the 1947 act detail precautions relating to the sale and letting of dwellings. As all the specified infectious diseases are, by article 7 of the 1981 regulations, excluded from the application of these sections of the act, these sections have no application at present. Section 37, relating to infectious premises notices is linked to these sections.

Detention and isolation of persons

Under section 38 (as amended by section 35 of the 1953 act), a chief medical officer, with the agreement of a second medical practitioner, may order the detention of a person who is a probable source of infection in a hospital or other place. Safeguards, including an appeal to the minister, are written into the section. It could be used only in the case of acute anterior poliomyelitis, cholera, diphtheria, plague, smallpox, tuberculosis, typhoid and paratyphoid, typhus and viral haemorrhagic diseases (including lassa fever and marburg disease) (article 8 of 1981 regulations).

Burial of body of person dying from an infectious disease

Under section 39 of the 1947 act, a health board may arrange for the burial of a person dying in an institution from an infectious disease, or may contribute towards the cost where the remains are buried in a place not near the deceased's place of residence. Under article 12 of the 1981 regulations, medical officers of health have duties 'with regard to the custody, transport and disposal of the

211

body of a person which is a probable source of infection with an infectious disease'.

Accommodation for persons compelled to leave home
Section 40 gives health boards authority to provide accomodation for persons 'compelled to leave their homes on account of any steps taken under this Act or the regulations made thereunder for the prevention of the spread of infectious disease'.

Rehabilitation
Section 41 of the 1947 act gave power to health authorities to arrange a rehabilitation service for 'persons suffering or recovering from an infectious disease'. This section was repealed by the Health Act, 1953 and replaced by section 50 of that act, which provided for a rehabilitation service for disabled persons generally.

Nursing services
Section 42 of the 1947 act allowed health authorities to provide 'nurses for attendance on persons suffering from infectious disease' either free or at a charge. At present, this power would seem to be complemented by section 60 of the Health Act, 1970, which deals with home nursing generally.

Presumption in civil actions
Section 43 provides that where a civil action arises out of one person being infected through another not taking the precautions prescribed, the court will assume that the latter was the cause of the infection being spread unless he can prove that the circumstances were such that it was unlikely that his failure to take the precautions led to the other person getting the disease.

Maintenance allowances
A scheme of maintenance allowances for persons suffering from infectious disease and persons who are probable sources of infection was introduced under section 44 of the 1947 act. It applies to acute anterior poliomyelitis, diphtheria, dysentery, salmonellosis, tuberculosis, typhoid and paratyphoid, typhus and viral haemorrhagic diseases (including lassa fever and marburg disease). The conditions for qualifying for these allowances are specified in section 44. The minister has power to make regulations governing the rates of payment. He has used this power since the introduction of the scheme

212

and the rates have been revised regularly.

Subsection (7) of section 44 was repealed by the Health Services (Financial Provisions) Act, 1947 (No 47 of 1947) and subsections (4) and (8) by the Health Act, 1953.

Treatment of infectious diseases in specified institutions
Under section 45 of the 1947 act, the minister 'may by order prohibit either absolutely or subject to specified conditions the admission of persons suffering from a specified infectious disease to, and the treatment of such persons in', any institution or part of an institution except one considered by the minister to be specially fitted for such treatment.

Verminous persons and articles
Sections 46 to 50 of the 1947 act deal with precautions to be taken relating to infestation by vermin (vermin being defined as 'any insects, being bugs, fleas, lice or itch mites'). Section 49 gives the minister power to make regulations on precautions to be taken in establishments from which there is an especial danger of the spread of infestation. No such regulations have been made.

Role of health boards
Under article 10 of the 1981 regulations, a health board has the duty to 'make arrangements for the diagnosis and treatment of infectious diseases in persons in the functional area of that health board'. The article specifies that no charge may be made for such services, except where provided in a private or semi-private ward or where the services are otherwise of a type for which it is customary to make an extra charge. It is also made clear that this article does not affect any agreement with an authority in another state for making payments to health boards for the treatment of infectious diseases.

Under article 13, health boards are required to keep supplies of diagnostic and prophylactic agents, instruments and equipment and to arrange for the administration of such agents. The boards may also make supplies of such agents available to medical practitioners.

Under article 20, a health board is required to keep such records as may be directed by the minister from time to time in relation to the exercise of its powers and the performance of its duties under the regulations. There are provisions in the article on keeping these records confidential:

Duties of medical officers of health, etc.
Article 11 of the 1981 regulations states:
> On becoming aware, whether from a notification or intimation under these regulations or otherwise, of a case or a suspected case of infectious disease or a probable source of infection with such disease, a medical officer of health, or a health officer on the advice of a medical officer of health, shall make such enquiries and take such steps as are necessary or desirable for investigating the nature and source of such infection and for removing conditions favourable to such infection.

A medical officer of health is defined as 'a director of community care and medical officer of health, the Dublin Medical Officer of Health, or any senior area medical officer or area medical officer of a health board' and 'health officer' is defined as 'an officer of a health board authorised by the health board to enforce any provisions of these regulations' (article 2). Duties relating to bodies of deceased people are referred to above.

Under article 18, a medical officer of health is required to make weekly returns to the minister of cases of infectious disease notified to him and to make detailed reports on cases of specified infectious diseases.

NOTIFICATIONS BY MEDICAL PRACTITIONERS

Article 14 requires a medical practitioner, 'as soon as he becomes aware or suspects that a person on whom he is in professional attendance is suffering from or is the carrier of an infectious disease' to send a written notification to the medical officer of health. Where it is a case of poliomyelitis, bacterial meningitis, cholera, ornithosis, plague, smallpox, typhus, a viral haemorrhagic disease, or yellow fever, he is required to give immediate preliminary notification.

Where a case of infectious disease is first diagnosed specifically in an infectious disease hospital or unit, or where a suspected case is admitted and the suspicion is not confirmed the medical officer in the hospital is required to make a notification to the medical officer of health (article 15). Fees for notifications by medical practitioners are payable by the health board under article 17.

Duty of registrars of births and deaths
Article 16 states:
>A registrar of births and deaths shall send to a medical officer of health such returns of deaths from infectious diseases as may be specified by the Minister.

INTERNATIONAL HEALTH REGULATIONS

Under the International Health Regulations, which were adopted by the World Health Organisation in 1951, each member state of the organisation is obliged to take steps to keep the organisation informed of the occurrence of outbreaks of plague, cholera, smallpox or yellow fever and to take steps to prevent these diseases from spreading to other countries. The regulations oblige the health administrations to provide at ports and airports the facilities necessary for taking the prescribed measures to prevent the diseases referred to from spreading. The maximum steps which any member state of the World Health Organisation may take with the aim of protecting its territory against the diseases are delimited. Sanitary measures must be completed without unnecessary delay to traffic and must be carried out so as not to cause undue discomfort to any person, or injury to health, and not to damage the structure of ships or aircraft. What may be done by the local health authorities in respect of departing and arriving vessels and aircraft is specified in considerable detail, as are the measures which may be taken in respect of each of the diseases covered by the regulations.

These regulations have been accepted by most member states of the organisation. The Irish health regulations governing sea and air traffic, mentioned above and the administrative practices under them are in conformity with the International Health Regulations.

APPENDIX C

Notes on laws on food and drugs

These notes are a guide to the legal provisions operative on 1 January 1988 but anyone needing a precise detailed knowledge of them should refer to the legal texts and any changes made hereafter in them.

The law on these matters is contained in part V and section 65 of the Health Act, 1947 (as amended), the Sale of Food and Drugs Acts 1875 to 1936, the Poisons (Ireland) Act, 1870, the Poisons and Pharmacy Act, 1908, the Therapeutic Substances Act, 1932 (No 25 of 1932) the Poisons Act, 1961, (No 12 of 1961), the Misuse of Drugs Acts 1977 and 1984, the Control of Chemical Trials Act, 1987 (No 28 of 1987) and the several sets of regulations made under these acts mentioned below.

THE FOOD HYGIENE REGULATIONS

The Food Hygiene Regulations, 1950 to 1971, were made under section 54 of the Health Act, 1947 and section 55 of that act, as amended by section 38 of the Health Act, 1953.

The purpose of these regulations is to prohibit and prevent the sale of diseased or contaminated food and to prescribe hygienic precautions for the manufacture, preparation, sale and serving of food. 'Food' in the context of the regulations includes 'every article used for food or drink by man, other than drugs or water' and also includes ingredients of foods, flavouring or colouring matters, preservatives and condiments (section 53 of Health Act, 1947). The penalty for breaking the regulations may be a fine of £100, with £10 a day for a continuing offence, or imprisonment for a term up to six months, or both fine and imprisonment.

Sale, etc. of unfit food
There is a general prohibition on the sale of unfit food, in the following terms:

> No person shall sell or offer or keep for sale:—
> (a)   any article of food intended for human consumption,
> (b)   any food animal or
> (c)   any food material
> which is diseased, contaminated or otherwise unfit for human consumption (article 9 of 1950 regulations).

This is supplemented by a provision making it an offence to sell or use in the manufacture or preparation of food any food or ingredient known to have been exposed to infection with a scheduled infectious disease (see article 10 of and the second schedule to the 1950 regulations. The scheduled infectious diseases are: acute anterior poliomyelitis, diphtheria, dysentery, salmonella infection, scarlet fever, streptococcal sore-throat, tuberculosis, typhoid and paratyphoid.)

Here it is as well to say that the terminology of the food hygiene regulations is based on a considerable number of interlocking artificial definitions (see article 2 of the 1950 regulations). 'Food animal' and 'food material' are among these definitions. The former means a dead farm animal (which animals are in turn defined as 'cattle, sheep, pigs, goats and poultry as defined in the Agricultural Produce (Fresh Meat) Act, 1930') or any other animal, whether living or dead, intended for food for human consumption. 'Food material' means 'any material or article which is used or intended for use in the preparation or manufacture of food intended for human consumption and which may enter into the composition of food'. These two definitions are cited because this is necessary for the comprehension of the important provisions referred to in the preceding paragraph. There are, however, no less than forty definitions of this nature in the regulations and it would not be possible to follow the intricacies of all of these in explaining what is contained in the rest of the regulations.

Seizure of unfit food
An 'authorised officer' (generally a health inspector or veterinary officer) may seize, remove and detain food, food animals or food material which he suspects to be diseased, contaminated or otherwise unfit for human consumption. Where this is done, the

article or animal may be destroyed there and then if the owner or person in charge agrees; if he does not, destruction or other disposal is contingent on an order of a district justice or a peace commissioner (article 11 of 1950 regulations). The provisions relating to the sale of unfit food do not, in general, apply to a number of agricultural products such as milk and pigs, where they are controlled under legislation administered by the Department of Agriculture and Food. The power to seize, remove and detain and the prohibition on transactions in food exposed to infection apply, however, to these products in the same way as to other foods.

Importation of unfit food (Chapter II of Part II of the 1950 regulations)
An importer of any food, food animal or food material who discovers that it is diseased, contaminated or otherwise unfit for human consumption, must so inform the local medical officer (or, in the case of cereals, a cereals officer of the Department of Agriculture and Food), do what that officer directs as to where and how it may be stored and, in accordance with the specification of the officer, destroy, re-export, re-condition or otherwise deal with it. Where the medical officer (or the cereals office) has advance information to the effect that an article of food, food animal or food material is unfit for human consumption, he may make an order prohibiting its importation or, where it has been landed, its removal from the place of importation. There is an appeal to a district justice or a peace commissioner against such an order. There are special controls on the importation of meat. The prohibitions and controls on import in the regulations do not apply to posted articles or to food in the personal baggage of the importer. Neither do they apply to food, food animals or food material for consumption on a vehicle, ship or aircraft.

Powers of inspection, sampling, etc. (Chapter III of Part II of the 1950 regulations)
Enforcing officers have wide powers of inspection and those in charge of food or food businesses must facilitate them in their inspections. Samples of food, materials used in preparing food or by-products of food manufacture may be taken without payment by the medical officer or other authorised officer and where a sample has been taken, the officer may direct a standstill on movement of the consignment until the result of the test on the sample is known. Persons carrying on food businesses must give the

authorised officer all reasonable assistance and information, including information on the origin and destination of their purchases and sales (retail traders however would not be expected to record the names of the purchasers of their goods).

Control of manufacture, retail trade, etc. (Part III of the 1950 regulations)
With the exception of food processes and transactions controlled by the Department of Agriculture and Food under its legislation, all manufacture, preparation, handling, serving, selling and transport of food is subject to control under the Food Hygiene Regulations. Over twenty different 'shalls' and 'shall-nots' are set out for the proprietors of food premises, ranging from a requirement for the 'walls, ceilings, floors, doors, windows and all parts of the premises' to be 'kept in a proper state of repair and in a clean and hygienic condition' to the exclusion of cats and dogs (except in certain circumstances). Ventilation, lighting, water supply, washing facilities, drainage, sanitary accommodation and refuse disposal are also covered. Machinery must be 'constructed and adjusted so as to prevent the contamination of food or food material by dirt from the mechanism' and chipped or cracked ware may not be used to serve food. Precautions must be taken against the contamination of food 'by foreign matter or unnecessary handling or by rats, mice or insects or otherwise' and unsuitable wrapping materials are barred. To complement these and the other specific prohibitions, article 25 of the regulations concludes by requiring the proprietor of the food premises to 'take every other reasonable precaution to prevent danger to the public health arising from the food business and to prevent the contamination of food in the food premises'.

Stalls and vehicles from which food is sold are required to comply with similar conditions and those selling food 'otherwise than at a food premises or a food stall' (such as those carrying it in a box or basket) are also governed by the regulations. Vehicles in which food is transported must be properly constructed and kept clean and, in their use, adequate steps must be taken to prevent the contamination of food. Containers in which food is carried must also be properly constructed and cared for and food ready to be eaten (such as bread) must be carried in a covered container.

Each worker in a food business is required to keep himself clean, to keep the equipment he uses in a clean and hygienic condition, to refrain from doing anything to contaminate the food on which he works and generally to take all reasonable precautions to prevent danger to the public health arising from his work. Visitors to places where food is being prepared must observe like precautions.

A person likely to cause infection with any of the scheduled infectious diseases (see page 210) or who has a boil, septic sore or other skin ailment on the hand or forearm which could contaminate food may not work in a food business except with the permission of the local medical officer. The proprietor must ask anyone who intends to take up employment in a food business whether he is a probable source of infection with a scheduled infectious disease or whether he ever suffered from typhoid or paratyphoid. The person seeking employment must answer this question to the best of his knowledge.

All these requirements may seem to place those in the food business in continuous danger of prosecution. In fact, however, many of the provisions are such as would be observed in any event by decent and competent manufacturers and dealers. Furthermore, health inspectors endeavour in the first place to educate food traders to observe the regulations. Prosecution is not resorted to for all violations and, generally speaking, an offender will be brought to court only where there is deliberate and dangerous violation of the code of food hygiene.

To deal with a case where there is a grave and immediate danger to public health from conditions in a premises or vehicle or at a stall, the minister has power to make an order directing the immediate cessation of the use of the premises, vehicle or stall for the purposes of a food business. There is an appeal to the district justice against such an order.

Registration of food premises (Part IV of 1950 regulations, as amended by the Food Hygiene (Amendment, Regulations, 1971)

Registration of all the premises to which the provisions mentioned under the preceding heading apply is provided for but the scheme of registration can be applied piecemeal by minister's order to different areas and different classes of premises. Hotels, holiday camps and restaurants and fishmongers', poulterers', butchers', pork butchers', ice-cream makers', manufacturers' and wholesalers' premises became registrable under the Food Hygiene Regulations, 1950 (Commencement of Part IV) Order, 1951 (S.I. No. 270 of 1951). 'Take away' food premises became registrable under the Food Hygiene Regulations Order 1986 (S.I. No 21 of 1986). When registration is applied to any type of premises, there follows a period of a year during which proprietors apply for registration, the health board tells each one if any alterations to the premises are called for and any such alterations can be made. The requirement to be registered becomes effective at the end of the year and before then the health board will have dealt with each application by registering the premises, granting provisional registration for a period up to six months, or refusing registration on stated grounds. At the end of the period for which it is granted, provisional registration can be made no longer provisional, can be withdrawn, or can be extended for one more period.

There is an appeal to the minister against a decision of the chief executive officer of a health board not to register a premises and, for those who were in business when registration was ordained for the particular class of premises, a further appeal lies to a district justice. After the expiration of the year of grace, no one can carry on a food business of a type specified in the commencement order in a premises which is not registered. Persons wishing to start any such businesses thereafter should apply for and obtain registration before they commence to operate.

Registration attaches to the premises and not to the proprietor. When a business changes hands, the health board merely alters the name in their register.

Where a registered proprietor of a food premises is convicted of an offence under Part III of the regulations, the health board is called upon to see during the following year whether the neglect to comply with this part of the regulations continues. If it does, the board may ask the minister to order the cancellation of the registration. When so asked (or when satisfied from enquiries initiated by himself) the minister may make an order cancelling or suspending registration.

An appeal to annul any such order may be made to the district justice.

An occasional food premises (defined in article 2 of the 1950 regulations as 'a food premises in which a food business is carried on for not more than two months at any time and for not more than four months in any calendar year) is not subject to the full requirements of registration. Special permits are issued by health boards for each occasional use of a premises.

Hygiene of ice-cream (Part V of 1950 regulations, as amended by the 1961 and 1971 regulations)

To supplement the general provisions of the regulations, there are special requirements in the preparation of ice-cream. 'Heat-treatment' of the mix, or the use of safe ingredients, is prescribed and the temperatures at which the mix be kept before being made into ice-cream are specified. Frequent recordings of temperatures are required in the making and storing of ice-cream and suitable thermometers must be installed for this purpose.

Shellfish (Part VI of 1950 regulations)

To avoid typhoid being transmitted by bivalve shellfish (oysters, clams, cockles, mussels or similar shellfish) or periwinkles taken from areas which might be polluted by sewage, the sale of these shellfish is controlled. Purification of such shellfish by an approved method before sale is required where they have been taken from a 'controlled area' (The controlled areas (which adjoin parts of the coasts of Cork, Galway, Kerry, Louth, Mayo, Sligo, Waterford and Wexford) are specified in the Food Hygiene Regulations, 1950 (Shellfish Controlled Areas) Orders, 1951, 1952, 1971, 1977 and 1984. Persons dealing in shellfish must keep records of where the fish come from and, except for retailers, to whom they are sold.

SALE OF FOOD AND DRUGS ACTS

The Sale of Food and Drugs Acts 1875 to 1936 were designed to prevent the sale of food or drugs which are injurious to health or 'not of the nature, substance and quality demanded by the purchaser'. Food and drugs inspectors are appointed by the health boards. These are mainly health inspectors. Public analysts are employed by the health boards to report on samples taken under the acts.

A food and drugs inspector (or any other person who wishes to do so at his own expense) may purchase a sample of any food or drug and submit it for analysis. The sample is first divided in three. One part is sent for analysis, another is given to the vendor (who must be told that the sample is to be analysed) and the third part is kept by the inspector for future comparison. The court, where proceedings are taken under the act, may order this part of the sample to be sent to the State Chemist, as referee. Proceedings are normally taken by the inspector who took the sample.

Special provisions are included in respect of milk, butter and margarine. Milk is regarded as not being of the 'nature, substance and quality' demanded by the purchaser if it does not contain prescribed percentages of milk-fat and other milk solids. Similar provisions relate to cream, buttermilk and skimmed milk. The percentages are prescribed in the Milk (Percentages of Milk-fat and Milk-solids) (No. 2) Regulations, 1936 (S.R. & O 321). They are: for milk 3% milk fat and 8.5% other milk solids; for cream 25% milk fat; for skimmed milk 8.6% milk solids not fat and for buttermilk 6.2% milk solids not fat. Butter or margarine may not contain more than 16% of water. Margarine may not contain more than 10% of butter fat and its wrapper must also be conspicuously marked so as to distinguish it from butter.

FOOD STANDARDS

The Minister for Health, if of the opinion that the composition of any food is of special importance to the public health, may, under section 56 of the Health Act, 1947, as amended by section 38 of the 1953 act, prescribe a standard for the chemical composition of that food. The only standard so far laid down in the exercise of this power is that for ice-cream. This standard was fixed by the Food Standards (Ice-cream) Regulations, 1952 (S.I. No 227 of 1951). It requires at least 5% milk fat, 9% other milk solids and 10% sugar (by weight in each case) in ice-cream. In addition to the powers conferred on him under the Health Act, 1947, the Minister for Health is also empowered, under the Food Standards Act, 1974, to prescribe standards for food but has not used this power.

Regulation of additives in food
The use of additives in food (preservatives, colouring agents, antioxidants and solvents) and the presence of undesirable substances such as lead and mineral hydrocarbons in food are controlled by regulations under the Health Acts 1947, 1953 and 1970 and the European Communities Act, 1972 (No 27 of 1972). The current regulations are:

Health (Cyclamate in Food) Regulations, 1970 (S.I. No 49 of 1970)
Health (Sampling of Food) Regulations, 1970 (S.I. No. 50 of

1970)

Health (Arsenic and Lead in Food) Regulations, 1972 (S.I. No. 44 of 1972)

Health (Mineral Hydrocarbons in Food) Regulations, 1972 (S.I. No 45 of 1972)

Health (Solvents in Food) Regulations, 1972 (S.I. No. 304 of 1972)

Health (Antioxidant in Food) Regulations, 1973 (S.I. No. 148 of 1973)

Health (Antioxidant in Food) (Amendment) Regulations, 1983 (S.I. No 61 of 1983)

European Communities (Antioxidant in Food) (Purity Criteria) Regulations, 1985 (S.I. No. 187 of 1985). (EC Council Directive 78/664)

Health (Colouring Agents in Food) Regulations, 1973 (S.I. No. 149 of 1973)

Health (Colouring Agents in Food) (Amendment) Regulations, 1981 (S.I. No. 336 of 1981)

Health (Erucic Acid in Food) Regulations, 1978 (S.I. No. 123 of 1978)

European Communities (Erucic Acid in Food) (Method of Analysis) Regulations, 1982 (S.I. No. 271 of 1982) (EC Council Directive 80/89)

Health (Emulsifiers, Stabilisers, Thickening and Gelling Agents in Food) Regulations, 1980 (S.I. No. 35 of 1980)

Health (Emulsifiers, Stabilisers, Thickening and Gelling Agents) (Amendment) Regulations, 1982 (S.I. No. 273 of 1982)

Health (Emulsifiers, Stabilisers, Thickening and Gelling Agents in Food) (Amendment) Regulations, 1985 (S.I. No. 186 of 1985)

Health (Preservatives in Food) Regulations, 1981 (S.I. No. 337 of 1981)

European Communities (Preservatives in Food) (Purity Criteria) Regulations, 1981 (S.I. No. 184 of 1981) (EEC Council Directives 65/66, 67/428 and 76/463)

Health (Foods for Particular Nutritional Uses) Regulations, 1982 (S.I. No. 272 of 1982) (EC Council Directive 77/94)

European Communities (Food Additives) (Purity Criteria Verification) Regulations, 1983 (S.I. No. 60 of 1983) (EC Council Directive 81/712)

Health (Vinyl Chloride in Food) Regulations, 1984 (S.I. No 95 of 1984)

European Communities (Vinyl Chloride in Food) (Method of Analysis) Regulations, 1984 (S.I. No. 92 of 1984) (EC Council Directive 81/432)

POISONS

The Poisons Act, 1961 is largely an enabling act. The regulations made by the minister under section 14 of that act contain most of the current law on the sale of poisons and related matters. These are the Poisons Regulations, 1982 (S.I. No 188 of 1982) and the Poisons (Amendment) Regulations, 1986 (S.I. No 424 of 1986).

Specification of poisons
Under article 5 of the 1982 regulations, substances listed in the First Schedule are declared to be poisons. Over 800 substances (with salts, derivates etc added in some cases) are included in this schedule. It is divided into two parts.

Restrictions on sale of poisons
These are contained in article 6 of the 1982 regulations (as amended by the 1986 regulations), which reads:

6.(1) Subject to the provisions of these regulations a person shall not in the course of a business sell or offer or keep for sale –
    (a)   any poison set out in Part I of the First Schedule unless he is a person keeping open shop for the dispensing or compounding of medical prescriptions or for the sale of poisons in accordance with the Pharmacy Acts, 1875 to 1977 and where the sale of any such poison is made it shall be effected by or under the supervision of an authorised person or a registered druggist, or
    (b)   any poison set out in Part II of the First Schedule unless –
        (i) he is a person keeping open shop for the dispensing or compounding of medical prescriptions or for the sale of poisons in accordance with the Pharmacy Acts, 1875 to 1977 and where the sale of any such poison is made it shall be effected by or under the supervision of an authorised person or a registered druggist, or

(ii) he is a person licensed by a health board under article 14 in respect of the premises on which the said poison is sold or offered or kept for sale and where the sale of any such poison is made it shall be effected by that person.

(2) A person shall not sell or offer or keep for sale any poison from a travelling shop, vehicle or automatic vending machine.

Licences issued by health boards under article 14 (sub-article (8) of which was amended by the 1986 regulations) 'have effect only as respects poisons set out in Part II of the First Schedule'. The licence is related to a specific premises, it ordinarily is in force for two years and a fee of £20 is payable for it. A health board may refuse a licence for reasons set out in sub-article (8), as amended and may cancel or suspend a licence. There is an appeal to the minister against a refusal, cancellation or suspension. Conditions are laid down in article 15 of the regulations (as amended by the 1986 regulations) for sales by licencees under article 14.

Labelling, records, wholesale dealing, storage, etc
Labelling of containers for poisons is governed by detailed provisions in article 7 of the 1982 regulations. Article 8 deals with the keeping of books and records relating to sales of poisons (the present version of that article is contained in the 1986 regulations). This is supplemented by article 18 (as amended by the 1986 regulations) which requires further records of sales of certain highly dangerous poisons. Wholesale dealing in poisons is governed by article 9, storage by article 10, containers by article 11 and transport by article 12. Article 13 relates to distinctive colouring of pesticides. Article 16 contains special provisions on the sale of strychnine and article 17 relates to further restrictions on the sale and supply of certain poisons. Certain general exemptions from the regulations are set out in article 19.

Enforcement
The enforcement and execution of the regulations may be carried out by officers of the minister, by the Pharmaceutical Society of Ireland and its officers and, as respects their licences, health boards and their officers (article 20, as amended by the 1986 regulations). The powers of enforcers are specified in the article.

Appendix C

MEDICAL PREPARATIONS

Under section 65 of the Health Act, 1947 (as amended by section 39 of the Health Act, 1953 and section 36 of the Misuse of Drugs Act, 1977) the minister may 'make regulations for the control of the advertisement or sale of medical preparations or toilet preparations generally or of any specified class of such preparations or any particular medical preparation or toilet preparation'. The expression 'medical preparation' is defined as:

(a)   a substance which is sold under a proprietary designation and which may be used for the prevention or treatment of any human ailment, infirmity, injury or defect, or

(b)   any other prophylactic, diagnostic or therapeutic substance which may be used for the prevention or treatment of any human ailment, infirmity, injury or defect.

Subsection (3) specifies that the regulations can prohibit the 'manufacture, preparation, importation, distribution, sale or offering or keeping for sale' of a preparation 'either absolutely or subject to specified conditions', including the grant of a licence. It also allows for the control of advertising of medical preparations.

Medical Preparations (Advertisement and Sale) Regulations, 1958 (S.I. No. 135 of 1958)
These regulations, articles 2 and 6 of which were amended by the 1984 and 1987 regulations mentioned below, provide that medical preparations may not be publicly advertised in a manner that might lead to their use in the diagnosis, prevention or treatment in humans of certain scheduled ailments (such as cancer, tuberculosis and diabetes) and that all medical preparations on sale must contain a statement on the label or container thereof showing the detailed composition of the product and other specified information. (The advertisement of cures for venereal disease is prohibited by the Venereal Diseases Act, 1917).

Medical Preparations (Licensing, Advertisement and Sale) Regulations, 1984 (S.I. No 210 of 1984)
These regulations, which replaced the European Communities

227

(Proprietary Medicinal Products) Regulations, 1975, introduced a common statutory licensing system for all medical preparations, both proprietary and non-proprietary (i.e. generic). Under the regulations no person may put a new preparation on the market unless he holds a 'product authorisation' for it from the minister or is exempted under articles 5 or 12. The application of this licensing system to generic products which were on the market prior to 1 October, 1984, is being phased in, in accordance with the Second Schedule to the regulations, in the period up to 1 April, 1989.

In deciding on applications for product authorisations, the minister is advised by the National Drugs Advisory Board and takes into account the quality, safety and efficacy of the preparation. The regulations include provisions for revoking authorisations (article 9(2)). Authorisations are valid for five years unless previously revoked. Fees are charges in respect of applications (article 10).
(EC Council directives 65/65, 75/318, 75/319 and 83/570 relate to these regulations)

Manufacturers' and wholesalers' licences
The Medical Preparations (Licensing of Manufacture) Regulations, 1974 (S.I. No. 225 of 1974) and the Medical Preparations (Licensing of Manufacture (Amendment) Regulations 1975 (S.I. No. 302 of 1975) prohibit the manufacture of medical preparations except under a licence granted by the minister, with certain exemptions covering the day-to-day activities of doctors, dentists and pharmacists in dispensing for individual patients. The 1975 regulations brought the provisions of the earlier regulations into line with EC Council Directive 75/319, mainly in relation to the employment of qualified persons in manufacturing units.

Under the Medical Preparations (Wholesale Licences) Regulations, 1974 (S.I. No. 333 of 1974), the sale or supply of medical preparations by wholesale, with specified exceptions, requires a licence from the minister. Such a licence ordinarily remains in force for three years unless previously revoked. Fees are chargeable for these licences.

Control of Clinical Trials Act, 1987
The purpose of the Control of Clinical Trials Act, 1987 is to provide for a statutory system of control on clinical trials which involve the testing of drugs or other substances on individuals. This

system will replace an existing voluntary arrangement for the clearance of such trials through the National Drugs Advisory Board.

Under section 3 of the act, it will be necessary to make prior application to the minister for permission to conduct a trial and this section sets out details on the making of such applications. Under section 4 the minister must, after consulting the National Drugs Advisory Board, either grant or refuse permission within twelve weeks of the application being made. Section 5 allows for later variations in the trial with the minister's approval. Controls on the conducting of chemical trials are set out in section 6, section 7 deals with the revocation of permits by the minister and section 8 with the constitution and role of ethics committees set up for the conduct of chemical trials.

Section 9 sets out procedures for consent by participants in chemical trials. There are miscellaneous provisions in the remaining sections on the operation of the act, which will come into force when the minister has made an order for its commencement under section 19 and any necessary regulations under section 17.

Medical Preparations (Control of Sale) Regulations, 1987 (S.I. No. 18 of 1987)
The purpose of these regulations is to apply an up-to-date and comprehensive system of control to those medical preparations which should be supplied only against a prescription issued by a registered medical practitioner or registered dentist. The regulations provide that the prescription-only requirement will apply to the following medical preparations —

—those which are or which contain substances listed in the First Schedule to the regulations (subject to exemptions related to certain things, such as the manner of administration, use, dosage level, strength),
—those intended for use by means of parenteral administration,
—those which are or which contain new drug substances placed on the market in this country for the first time.

The control system provided for in respect of prescription-only medical preparations includes the following:

Restrictions in relation to the dispensing of prescriptions
These are set out in article 6. The extent of the restriction is based on whether the drug substance contained in the medical preparation in question is in Part A or Part B of the First

Schedule. Prescriptions for Part A preparations may, unless otherwise directed, be dispensed on one occasion only. Medical preparations containing new drug substances and injectables are treated likewise. Prescriptions for Part B preparations may, unless otherwise directed, be dispensed as often as the pharmacist deems appropriate within a period of six months from the date of issue of the prescription.

No prescription for a prescription-only medical preparation may be dispensed after the end of the period of six months from the date of the prescription.

Labelling requirements
These are set out in article 8 and provide for the mandatory labelling of all dispensed medical preparations. They must be labelled with the warning 'keep out of the reach of children' and where a preparation is for external use the words 'for external use only'.

Pharmacy record-keeping
These requirements are set out in article 9. They place an obligation on the pharmacist to keep for a period of two years a register of the particulars included on each prescription dispensed and, except in the case of a repeatable prescription, the prescription. Provision is also made for the acceptance of computer records in place of the register where a daily print-out certified by the managing pharmacist is kept for inspection.

Prohibition on advertising to the public
Article 10 of the regulations prohibits the advertising to the public of any prescription-only medical preparation.

Prohibition on sale after expiry date
Article 11 of the regulations prohibits the sale (including the keeping or offering for sale) of any medical preparation after its expiry date.

One of the principal features of the new controls is the level of professional discretion which is given to the pharmacist in relation to the supply of 'prescription-only' medical preparations in emergency situations . This particular aspect is dealt with in article 7 where the conditions under which a pharmacist may supply a medical preparation in such circumstances are specified.

The regulations may be enforced by officers of the minister, the Pharmaceutical Society and its officers and health boards and their officers.

Therapeutic Substances Act, 1932 (No 25 of 1932)
The Therapeutic Substances Act, 1932, applies to vaccines sera, toxins, antitoxins, antigens and certain other substances whether used in the treatment of human or animal disease. The general purpose of the act is to ensure that such substances, the purity and potency of which cannot be adequately tested by chemical means, will comply with certain standards of potency, quality and purity. The controls provide for the licensing of manufacture and importation. The sale of such substances is subject to requirements as to the type of container, labelling and compliance with conditions as to expiry dates, etc. The Therapeutic Substances Advisory Committee, a statutory body, advises and assists the minister in the operation of this act.

Pharmacopoeia Act, 1931 (No 22 of 1931)
This act recognised the British Pharmacopoeia for use as an Irish pharmacopoeia and medicines are accordingly compounded in accordance with it. Section 35 and 42 of the Misuse of Drugs Act, 1977 amended the 1931 act in some respects, including recognition of the European Pharmacopoeia which was prepared under the auspices of the Council of Europe in 1964.

MISUSE OF DRUGS

Dangerous or otherwise harmful drugs are controlled under the Misuse of Drugs Act, 1977 (No 12 of 1977) as amended and extended by the Misuse of Drugs Act, 1984 (No 18 of 1984).

Controlled drugs
The list of drugs controlled is in the schedule to the 1977 act. The list may be varied by government order under section 2 of the act. It has been varied by the Misuse of Drugs Act, 1977 (Controlled Drugs) (Declaration) Order 1987 (S.I. No. 251 of 1987).

Possession of controlled drugs
Possession of controlled drugs is prohibited under section 3 of the

1977 act but the Misuse of Drugs (Exemption) Order, 1979 (S.I. No. 29 of 1979) as amended by the Misuse of Drugs (Exemption) (Amendment) Order, 1987 (S.I. No 264 of 1987) exempts from the prohibition a number of preparations in which there are but small quantities of controlled drugs. Further exemptions are detailed in Part III of the Misuse of Drugs Regulations, 1979 (S.I. No. 32 of 1979). Section 15 of the 1977 act relates to possession for the purpose of sale or supply to others.

Regulations to prevent misuse of drugs
Section 5 of the 1977 act gives the minister power to make regulations governing, among other things:

   (i) the manufacture, production or preparation of controlled drugs,
   (ii) the importation or exportation of controlled drugs,
   (iii) the supply, the offering to supply or the distribution of controlled drugs,
   (iv) the transportation of controlled drugs.

The relevant regulations are the Misuse of Drugs Regulations, 1979, as amended by the Misuse of Drugs (Amendment) Regulations, 1987 (S.I. No 263 of 1987), the Misuse of Drugs (Safe Custody) Regulations, 1982 (S.I. No. 321 of 1982), which replaced article 22 of the 1979 regulations, and the Misuse of Drugs (Designation) Order, 1979 (S.I. No. 30 of 1979).

Control of prescribing, supply, etc. in certain cases
Sections 6 to 12 of the 1977 act, as amended by sections 3 and 4 of the 1984 act, contain extensive provisions to deal with cases where it is thought that a practitioner (a doctor, a dentist or a veterinary surgeon) or a pharmacist is involved in certain abuses relating to controlled drugs.

The Misuse of Drugs (Committees of Inquiry) Regulations, 1984 (S.I. No. 264 of 1984) relate to this. Forgery of prescriptions is dealt with in section 18 of the 1977 act.

Opium and cannabis
Special provisions on these are contained in sections 16, 17 and 19 of the 1977 act, as amended by section 11 of the 1984 act.

Enforcement and penalties
Section 20 to 31 of the 1977 act, as amended and extended by sections 5 to 10 and 12 to 14 of the 1984 act relate to enforcement and penalties (which were substantially increased under the latter act). The Misuse of Drugs (Custodial Treatment Centre) Order, 1980 (S.I. No. 30 of 1980) designated the Central Mental Hospital at Dundrum, Dublin as a place where persons convicted of certain offences under the acts may receive custodial medical treatment or care.

COSMETICS

The European Communities (Cosmetic Products) Regulations, 1984 (S.I. No. 11 of 1984), as amended by the European Communities (Cosmetic Products) Regulations, 1986 (S.I. No 35 of 1986) and the European Communities (Cosmetic Products) (Amendment) Regulations, 1987 (S.I. No. 240 of 1987) give statutory effect to various EC directives relating to cosmetic products (EC Council Directives 76/78, 79/661, 80/1335, 82/147, 82/368, 82/434, 83/191, 83/341, 83/496, 83/514, 83/574, 84/415, 85/391, 85/490, 86/179, 86/199 and 87/137). The main thrust of the regulations is to prohibit the marketing of cosmetic products dangerous to health.

APPENDIX D

The general medical service

PART 1

THE PARTICIPATION OF MEDICAL PRACTITIONERS

General conditions
1. The conditions for participation in the service are specified in the agreement, which is in a prescribed form, between the health board and the medical practitioner.
2. The conditions for participation in the service (including fees) which have been agreed on between the minister and the medical profession relate only to a situation in which there is no significant change in the percentage of population eligible for the service.

Choice of doctor
3. Subject to what follows and to paragraph 6 below, an eligible person is allowed to register with any participating doctor who has not already got a list up to the maximum (see paragraph 10). His choice is, however, subject to the condition that the doctor does not live more than seven miles from the patient, but this condition does not apply in certain individual cases, such as where there is no doctor within seven miles. Where the doctor wishes to take on a patient living more than seven miles from him and where other doctors practise within seven miles of the patient's residence, the domiciliary fee payable is that appropriate to a distance of seven miles.

Persons for whom doctor is responsible
4. The doctor is responsible for
(a) all eligible persons whom he has accepted for inclusion in his

list and who have not been notified to him by the board as having ceased to be on the list,

(b) all eligible persons assigned to him by the board in accordance with paragraph 5 below and who have not been notified to him by the board as having ceased to be on his list,

(c) all eligible persons whom he has accepted as temporary residents,

(d) all eligible persons in respect of whom he is acting as deputy to another practitioner,

(e) all eligible persons whom it is necessary for him to treat in an emergency situation.

5. The doctor may be assigned eligible persons by the board. In areas where there is a choice between doctors providing services for eligible persons the power of assignment by the board is used only in the case of persons who have unsuccessfully applied to a number of doctors for acceptance on their lists. The assignment of a patient is to the nearest doctor unless there is a valid contradication, but assignments are reviewed at reasonable intervals. In areas where the choice of another doctor is impossible or impracticable, the doctor is obliged to accept on his list all eligible patients in that area who seek inclusion in his list. In the exceptional case where a group of patients more than ten miles from a doctor is assigned to him there is a special allowance for this responsibility in addition to the scheduled fees. The amount of the allowance is related to the number of patients and the distance involved and is negotiated with the Irish Medical Organisation.

6. The doctor is not required to provide services for any person whom he is unwilling to accept as a patient unless the person concerned is one assigned to him by the board or unless he is called upon to attend the patient in an emergency situation.

Temporary residents

7. A temporary resident is an eligible person who temporarily moves into a district not served by the doctor in whose list he is included and who does not, at the time of his arrival in the district, intend to remain there for a period exceeding three months. If his stay within the district extends to more than three months, his residence shall as from the end of that period cease to be regarded as temporary.

Itinerant families

8. Health boards, through their own officers or through voluntary organisations, ensure that eligible itinerant families are issued with medical cards and are accepted on the lists of doctors in the areas where the itinerants are normally resident. Where itinerant families move outside these areas they are regarded as temporary residents.

Unregistered children

9. Where a doctor is requested to provide a service for a young child whose name has not already been added to the list of dependants covered by the family registration, he shall provide the service and claim the appropriate fee on a specially prescribed form.

Limitation on numbers

10. The normal limit to the number of eligible persons on the doctor's list is 2,000 but in exceptional cases, the board may decide not to apply this limit.

Discontinuance of acceptance of a person

11. A doctor wishing to discontinue his acceptance of an eligible person, other than a person assigned by the board, may do so on giving notice to the board. If the doctor informs the board of his desire to discontinue his acceptance of an eligible person, the board notifies the person accordingly and supplies him with a notice enabling him to apply to another doctor. The person's name is removed from the doctor's list as from the date on which the doctor receives intimation that the person has been accepted by or assigned to another doctor.

Change of doctor

12. Where a person whose name is included in the list of a doctor wishes to transfer to the list of another doctor he applies on a prescribed form to the health board seeking such transfer. The name of the other doctor is specified in the application and it is a matter for the person to seek from him acceptance of the transfer and for the doctor to indicate such acceptance on the application form. The first doctor ceases to be responsible for the patient on the date he receives a notification from the health board that the patient has been transferred to another list.

Manner of providing service

13. The doctor is obliged to render to his patients all proper and necessary treatment of a kind usually undertaken by a general medical practitioner and not requiring special skill or experience of a degree or kind which general practitioners cannot reasonably be expected to possess.

14. The doctor undertakes to be available for consultation at his surgery (surgeries) for a specified number of hours weekly and to be available for consultation and for domiciliary visiting for an aggregate of forty hours weekly during normal hours. He also undertakes to have suitable arrangements to enable contact with him outside normal hours for emergency cases.

15. Where a doctor chooses to arrange some routine surgery hours or to do some of his routine domiciliary calls outside normal working hours he is not entitled to claim more than the normal fee for these services.

16. The doctor undertakes to maintain his surgery (surgeries) in a suitable condition for the purposes of his medical practice and, if required, to allow inspection by a representative of the board for the purposes of establishing its (their) suitability.

17. Surgery arrangements made by the doctor may not discriminate between eligible persons and the practitioner's private patients.

Obtaining 'second opinions'

18. Subject to such conditions or directions as the minister may lay down from time to time following consultation with the medical organisations a doctor may when he considers it desirable have a consultation with another medical practitioner in regard to an eligible patient on his list and the health board is liable for the cost of such consultation.

Prescribing and dispensing

19. The doctor is obliged to prescribe on the official prescription form such drugs and appliances as he considers necessary for the eligible person and in doing so he must act in accordance with any administrative requirements as to the completion of the form. While nothing in these requirements may interfere with the practitioner's discretion as to the amount and nature of the items prescribed, it is expected that doctors will bear in mind the need for economy. Where the prescribing pattern of a medical practitioner appears to be abnormal the circumstances may be investigated by a medical officer acting on behalf of the General Medical Services (Payments)

Board. If the medical officer so decides the circumstances may then be referred for consideration by an investigating committee referred to in paragraph 50.

20. The doctor shall supply to a person on his list such drugs and appliances as the doctor shall consider necessary for immediate administration or application. Where the doctor is not a dispensing doctor he may recoup from a retail pharmacist who has an agreement with the health board, the items so supplied by giving to him on the prescribed form a 'prescription' in the name of the patient or patients.

21. Subject to paragraphs 22 and 25, dispensing under the scheme is normally done by a retail pharmacist.

22. Where a doctor has only one centre of practice and it is three miles or more from the nearest retail pharmacist all patients on the doctor's list are asked to indicate whether they wish to have their prescriptions dispensed by the doctor or by a retail pharmacist. To remunerate him for his services a doctor is paid an annual fee in respect of each patient who opts to have his prescriptions dispensed by the doctor.

23. Where a doctor has a number of centres of practice, one or more within three miles of a pharmacy and one or more over three miles from a pharmacy only those patients who would normally be expected to attend the distant centre have a right to opt for dispensing by the doctor.

24. When a pharmacist opens a pharmacy within three miles of a dispensing doctor's centre of practice his eligible patients cease to have a choice between the doctor and the pharmacist for dispensing purposes. As from a date to be determined by the health board these patients may have their prescriptions dispensed by the pharmacist (subject to paragraph 25).

25. Where a doctor lives within three miles of a pharmacist but where in the view of the health board it would be a hardship on certain individual patients because of disability to obtain their prescriptions from a retail pharmacist the doctor may, in such instances, be required to dispense for the patients. The doctor is paid an annual dispensing fee for each of these patients.

26. A dispensing doctor is obliged to obtain his requirements of drugs for eligible persons from a pharmacist who has entered into an agreement with the health board, and to complete requisitions, returns of stock and such other records as may be required of him. The pharmacist would be one in the doctor's normal area of

238

practice or, if there was none in that area, a reasonably convenient pharmacist outside that area.

27. An eligible person receiving consultant out-patient care at a hospital is normally referred back to his general practitioner who issues him with a prescription for whatever medicines he may require. In the exceptional instance where the hospital doctor considers it essential that he should issue a prescription himself a sufficient quantity may be dispensed from hospital stocks to carry the patient over until he can attend his general practitioner.

Medical records
28. A doctor is obliged to comply with such directions or regulations as the Minister for Health may make from time to time after consultation with the medical profession in regard to the keeping of medical records.

29. When an eligible patient for whom the doctor has been responsible is transferred to the list of another doctor in the service the former doctor, subject to the consent of the patient, gives to the latter doctor a summary of the medical history and condition of the patient.

Locums
30. The doctor makes arrangements for the employment of a suitably qualified deputy during absences. The initial obligation to obtain a locum rests with the participating doctor but health boards co-operate in obtaining one. Where a doctor falls ill the health board, if requested, has the obligation to obtain a locum.

31. The payment of the deputy is a matter for the doctor except in the case of some former dispensary doctors where it is the board's responsibility to make such payment. A participating doctor who pays his locum gets an allowance as a contribution towards locum and other practice expenses.

Partnerships and group practice
32. Where two or more doctors proposing to enter into agreements with the board are in partnership or in group practice each has to enter into an individual agreement with the board and will have his individual list of eligible patients and will be responsible for them in the same way as if he were practising independently.

33. Where one partner or one member of a group practice provides treatment for an eligible person on another partner's list, he will

do so in the capacity of a locum tenens and he will not be entitled to claim an emergency fee or a temporary resident's fee for attending such a person.

34. The creation of a position as partner, or as an additional member of a group practice, or as an assistant with a view to partnership for the purpose of the general medical service, is subject to the approval of the health board. In considering any such proposal the board has regard to the total practice of the applicant. Before giving approval the board must be satisfied:—

(a) that the creation of the position is preferable to the creation of an additional position which could be filled by open competition in the normal way; and

(b) that the creation of the position will not result in the admission of a particular person into the general medical service while other equally well or better qualified persons are not given a reasonable chance to compete.

Where the chief executive officer proposes to seek the approval of the board to the creation of a position as a partner, or as an additional member of a group practice, or as an assistant with a view to partnership he shall, before doing so, consult the Irish Medical Organisation.

35. Where a health board agrees to the creation of a partnership or an addition to a group practice or to the recruitment of an assistant with a view to a partnership the position is advertised in the normal way but the doctor or doctors involved or a nominee of the doctor or doctors involved in the proposed taking in of a partner, or additional member or assistant is entitled to sit on the selection board. The selection board is obliged to pay due regard to any objection of this representative to the giving of the post to a particular individual or individuals. If the board considers it desirable it may not recommend any candidate for appointment.

Admission of doctors to the scheme

36. Ordinarily vacancies in the scheme are filled by public advertisement and interviews conducted by a board representative of the health board and the profession, with an independent chairman. Recruitment of doctors as partners or assistants with a view to partnership is based on panels of candidates set up by the health boards after similar advertisement and interviews. An assistant otherwise engaged by a participating doctor gets no right of access to the service.

37. In addition to the foregoing any doctor established in his own right in private practice in a particular centre for five years can become entitled to take public patients (but would not, of course, be given any guaranteed panel of such patients). Such a doctor would be entitled to apply to the health board for entry into the scheme and if he satisfies the board that he complied with the provision mentioned, he would be admitted to the scheme.

Qualifications
38. The minimum qualifications for doctors entering the service are two years' experience after full registration, six months of this being in general practice and the remainder being made up of three six-month periods of hospital experience in specified specialties.

Age limit
39. The contract of a participating doctor terminates when he reaches seventy years of age.

Remuneration
40. The rates of fees for surgery and domiciliary consultations and other payments to doctors are negotiated from time to time with the Irish Medical Organisation.
41. Where a doctor attends to more than one eligible patient in a household in the course of a domiciliary visit a fee at the appropriate domiciliary rate is payable for the first patient and a fee at the appropriate surgery rate for the other patient(s).
42. Where a doctor provides services from more than one centre of practice his fee for a domiciliary service is related to the distance the patient lives from the doctor's main centre of practice.
43. Where a doctor attends eligible persons in a home for the aged fees are payable on a sessional basis for routine visiting. The amount due to a doctor is calculated by totalling the number of hours spent by him each month in the routine visiting of eligible patients. The appropriate domiciliary fee is payable for non-routine calls to the home.
44. Where a doctor undertakes an urgent visit between 11 pm and midnight which necessarily involves his remaining on the call until after midnight he may claim the appropriate after-midnight fee for the service.
45. Where a doctor lives and practises in a centre with a population of less than 500 and where there is not a town with a population

of 1,500 or more within a three-mile radius of that centre the doctor may receive special rural practice concessions.

46. In these areas the doctor is paid full fees. In addition a rural practice allowance is payable:

(a) to a district medical officer with guarantees who opts to be paid on a fee basis,

(b) to any other participating practitioner who, at the commencement of the scheme, is entitled to participate in it and who is the sole participating practitioner in the centre in question,

(c) to any other participating practitioner if the health board decides to make this payment to retain him in the area.

47. For very remote areas, as specified by the minister, doctors may opt to be paid by fees or by salary or by a combination of fees and salary.

Medical certificates

48. The fees payable to the doctor cover the issue by him of certificates for such purposes as may be prescribed by the minister after consultation with the medical profession.

Submission and processing of claims for fees

49. Claims for payment are made to the General Medical Services (Payments) Board. Payments are processed by computer.

50. The computer maintains a continuing record of a doctor's visiting pattern. Where an instance of abnormal consultation is revealed the medical officer attached to the central unit seeks clarification from the doctor concerned. If there is evidence to suggest that the rate of consultation was not justified the medical officer reports the facts to an investigating committee consisting of a nominee of the minister, a representative of the organised profession and the medical officer acting on behalf of the central unit (not being the medical officer who investigated the circumstances).

51. The investigating committee decides whether the instance calls for no further action, for a warning, for a reduction in fees claimed or, in a serious case, for referral to the disciplinary tribunal referred to in paragraph 58. It is open to a doctor to appeal to the disciplinary tribunal against a decision of the committee. The form of agreement which doctors enter into with health boards includes a more detailed description of the provisions for penalties and the reduction of fees.

52. The doctor may not demand or accept any fee or other remuneration for services rendered to eligible persons other than the payment made to him under the agreement.

Practice premises

53. It is a condition of the practitioner's contract that on entry or by a specified date he has suitable premises available for his practice in which there will be common access to him by his eligible and private patients.

54. Health boards require participating doctors to provide and to continue to maintain the following facilities for patients:

(a) a waiting room with a reasonable standard of comfort, sufficient in size to accommodate the normal demands of his practice for both eligible and private patients and with adequate seating accommodation;

(b) a surgery sufficient in size for the requirements of normal general practice. Its facilities should include electric light, hot and cold running water, an examination couch and other essential needs of general practice;

(c) a telephone should be available for the doctor on the premises at the main centre of practice;

(d) toilet facilities should be accessible to patients.

A doctor is expected by the health board to give facilities for inspection of premises to establish suitability.

55. Health boards are empowered to give grants towards the provision of new practice premises or for the improvement or extension of the existing practice premises of participating doctors, ranging from 25% to 50% of the cost (subject to limits).

56. Participating doctors may be offered facilities to practise in existing health centres, dispensaries or other health board accommodation. Where a permanent district medical officer occupied a dispensary residence he is allowed to continue in occupation as long as he participates in the new service in the area concerned. Where a dispensary and residence are sited together only the doctor occupying the residence has a right to use that dispensary.

57. No charge is made to a former dispensary doctor with automatic right of participation, using a health centre, dispensary or other health board premises. An appropriate negotiated contribution towards running expenses is made by other practitioners availing of such facilities but they are provided free of charge for approved

partnerships or group practices.

Complaints against doctors

58. Complaints on the provision (or non-provision) of services by doctors are investigated in the first place by the staff of the health board. If the chief executive officer of the health board decides that a complaint is unfounded no further action is taken. If he decides that it is well-founded but relatively trivial, he has power to communicate with the doctor on the subject matter of the complaint. If the complaint appears on preliminary investigation to be of a serious nature the chief executive officer shall refer it to the disciplinary tribunal (a body set up under article 8 of the Health Services Regulations, 1972 (S.I. No. 88). It consists of a chairman selected in agreement with the medical profession and an even number of other members, of whom half are doctors appointed from a panel agreed with the profession).

59. The tribunal, having considered the complaint with all practicable speed may either:—

(a) dismiss it and let this dismissal be known to all concerned;

(b) uphold it and direct termination of the doctor's agreement;

(c) uphold it but recommend a lesser penalty by way of deduction of a specified sum from the doctor's remuneration or

(d) uphold it but decide that it is sufficient to admonish the doctor for his conduct.

60. There is an appeal to the minister against the termination of an agreement or other penalty recommended by the tribunal. On such an appeal the minister may uphold, modify or reverse the decision of the tribunal. This in no way cuts across normal rights of recourse to the courts.

Termination of agreement

61. A doctor may terminate his agreement on giving three months' notice, or such shorter notice as may be acceptable to the board.

62. The agreement shall be terminated forthwith where the medical practitioner's name is removed from the register of medical practitioners maintained by the Medical Council or where the disciplinary tribunal established to deal with complaints against medical practitioners participating in the service has so directed and after appeal, where made, the minister or the courts have upheld the decision.

63. The agreement shall be terminated on a doctor's taking up

wholetime employment outside the service.

64. The board may terminate the agreement where:

(a) the medical practitioner ceases to comply with the terms of the agreement, or

(b) the medical practitioner has been certified in accordance with a prescribed procedure to be discussed with the Irish Medical Organisation to be suffering from permanent infirmity of mind or body.

65. An appeal lies to the minister against the board's decision to terminate the agreement and, of course, the doctor also has a right of appeal to the courts.

PART II

SUPPLY OF DRUGS, MEDICINES AND APPLIANCES

Dispensing by pharmacists

1. The dispensing of drugs and medicines for an eligible person in the general medical service is normally done by a contracting pharmacist. The word pharmacist throughout this appendix means a registered pharmaceutical chemist or a registered dispensing chemist and druggist lawfully 'keeping open shop' in accordance with the provisions of the Pharmacy Acts 1875 to 1962.

2. When a pharmacist receives a prescription on an official form signed by a doctor he dispenses the items listed on the form. The items dispensed by the pharmacist should be entirely in accordance with the doctor's prescription unless the prescription contains obvious errors or omissions.

General conditions for participation of retail pharmacists

3. Every retail pharmacist is eligible for participation in the scheme provided he enters into the prescribed agreement with the relevant health board or health boards.

4. A pharmacist's agreement with a health board may be terminated by the board where it is satisfied that the pharmacist has failed to observe the terms of the agreement or that the pharmacist has been convicted of a criminal offence relating to the practice of pharmacy. The pharmacist may appeal to the minister against this termination.

5. A pharmacist's agreement with a health board shall automatically terminate upon the removal of his name from the register of the

Pharmaceutical Society of Ireland.

6. A pharmacist may terminate his agreement on giving three months' notice or such shorter notice as may be acceptable to the health board.

7. The conditions (including fees) for participation in the service which have been agreed relate only to a situation in which there will be no significant change in the percentage of population now eligible for the service.

Premises

8. A pharmacist is required to maintain satisfactory premises, equipment and stock and in this respect the premises may be inspected by an officer of the health board or of the General Medical Services (Payments) Board.

Hours of business

9. The pharmacist is obliged to keep his premises open for dispensing prescriptions during the hours specified in his agreement with the health board.

Basis of remuneration

10. The pharmacist is remunerated on the basis of the recoupment to him of the ingredient cost of prescription items dispensed for eligible patients under the scheme together with a fee for each item. The fee contains specific elements to cover the cost of containers, capital investment and obsolescence. Higher fees are paid for extemporaneous prescribing and for prescription items which involve the fitting of appliances. An additional fee is payable for urgent prescriptions dispensed outside contract hours.

11. The price of a proprietary item to the pharmacist is taken as the basic ex-wholesale price ruling during the month the prescription was dispensed. The ingredient cost of non-proprietary items is arrived at on the basis of agreed lists. A tariff is circulated to all pharmacists detailing the rates which are payable in respect of non-proprietary drugs, medicines and appliances. Manufacturing and wholesale firms notify the General Medical Services (Payments) Board of price changes in goods in advance of implementation. Pharmacists supplying dispensing doctors are reimbursed on the basis of the basic ex-wholesale price, with the addition of twenty-five per cent on cost.

Appendix D

Rates of remuneration

12. The rates of fees payable to pharmacists are negotiated from time to time with the Irish Pharmaceutical Union. The basic fee includes an element to recoup the pharmacist for the cost of obsolescence, capital investment and containers. Pharmacists are recouped value added tax paid by them in respect of supplies under the scheme.

Packs and containers

13. The size of pack from which pharmacists are expected to dispense prescriptions under the scheme is the size which would normally have a shelf life of one month having regard to the volume of business of the particular pharmacist. Where it appears that a pharmacist is dispensing from a smaller pack than is necessary and thereby increasing the ingredient cost of the item, the General Medical Services (Payments) Board seeks an explanation from the pharmacist and may make an appropriate deduction from payments due to him. Where, in order to meet the requirements of a particularly expensive prescription, a pharmacist is obliged to purchase a larger quantity than prescribed and where a portion of that pack remains on his hands after an agreed period, the full cost of the pack is paid to the pharmacist and the balance of the pack may be taken into stock by a health board pharmacy. Capsules, tablets, etc. should be dispensed in their original packs or in rigid containers. Containers made from paper board material are not acceptable.

Submission of claims for remuneration

14. A code book (with detailed instructions) covering drugs, medicines, dressings and appliances in common use is issued to each pharmacist. When a pharmacist dispenses a prescription he inserts on the prescription form the appropriate code number for each item dispensed. He also stamps and retains the form, which is in duplicate. If the prescription has been marked urgent by the doctor or certified urgent by the pharmacist and has been submitted to and dispensed by the pharmacist outside contract hours, he endorses it with the time of dispensing.

15. A pharmacist forwards all prescriptions dispensed by him under the scheme during a calendar month to reach the General Medical Services (Payments) Board not later than the seventh day of the following month. The period is extended to take account of any

247

public holidays. The pharmacist retains the duplicates of the prescriptions.

16. Payment to the pharmacist is normally made in full during the second half of the month following that in which the prescriptions are submitted. He receives with his payment cheque a detailed statement showing the manner in which the payment was calculated.

17. Where it is found that a prescription has been issued in error by a doctor to a person not eligible for participation in the scheme and the pharmacist has bona fide fulfilled the terms of the prescription, he is paid the appropriate amount for it.

APPENDIX E

Summary of provisions on mental treatment

These notes are a guide to the legal provisions operative on 1 January 1988 but anyone needing a precise detailed knowledge of them should refer to the legal texts and any changes made hereafter in them. Re the Health (Mental Services) Act, 1981, see footnote 1 to chapter nine.

The law on mental treatment is basically contained in the Mental Treatment Act, 1945 (No 19 of 1945) but that act has been amended and adapted on several occasions. The provisions in it on administration and eligibility have been superseded by the Health Acts and the 1945 act was otherwise amended in 1953 and 1961. Several technical adaptations in the provisions as they stood at that time were made by the Mental Treatment Acts (Adaptation) Order, 1971 (S.I. No 108 of 1971), to bring those provisions into conformity with the administrative changes effected by the Health Act, 1970. The main regulations under the Mental Treatment Acts are the Mental Treatment Regulations, 1961.

Modes of admission to mental hospitals
There are three categories in mental hospitals - voluntary patients, temporary patients and those certified as persons of unsound mind.

Reception orders for persons of unsound mind
An application to have a person received as being of unsound mind in a mental hospital is normally made by the husband, wife or other relative. Where the patient is in one of the classes entitled to use the health board's service and it is desired to have him admitted as such to the district mental hospital, the application is made to a medical practitioner. He examines the patient and, if satisfied, recommends that he be received in the district mental hospital.
Where such a recommendation has been made, the patient may

249

then be brought (with the assistance of an escort from the Garda Siochana if required for the safe conveyance of the patient) to the district mental hospital. The health board may co-operate with the applicant in making arrangements for the removal of the person to hospital. The person is then examined by the medical officer in charge or a deputy. If that officer is satisfied that the person should be received, he makes an 'eligible patient reception order'. This authorises the patient's detention in the mental hospital 'until his removal or discharge by proper authority or his death'.

Where the person is to be admitted as a private patient, whether to a district mental hospital or another mental hospital, the husband, wife or other relative may apply to any medical practitioner for a 'private patient reception order'. That medical practitioner arranges with a second medical practitioner to examine the patient separately and if both doctors are satisfied that it should be done, they make a reception order. This authorises the person in charge of the institution named in the order to receive and detain the patient.

Temporary patients

Mental hospitals and homes which are approved for that purpose by the Minister for Health may receive temporary patients. The admission and reception of such patients is governed by procedures similar to those for persons of unsound mind but the detention authorised is limited to a period of six months, except where this period is extended by the chief medical officer of the institution. Such an extension cannot be for more than six months at a time and the total period of detention of a temporary patient cannot exceed two years.

Detained persons - their rights, etc.

When the Inspector of Mental Hospitals visits a mental hospital he is required to give special attention to the state of mind of any detained person the propriety of whose detention he doubts or has been requested by the patient or another person to investigate. If he thinks that the patient's condition calls for it, the case is further examined and the minister may then direct the patient's discharge.

Detained persons may be allowed to be absent on trial for periods up to ninety days or on parole for periods up to forty-eight hours. They may also be boarded-out indefinitely in private dwellings, while remaining under surveillance by the medical staff of the mental hospital.

When a patient detained under a reception order recovers, his relatives are told and he is discharged. He cannot then be taken back into detention in a hospital except by the making of a fresh reception order.

There are several other safeguards contained in the Mental Treatment Acts against wrongful detention of patients. The principal ones are:

(a) Every patient has a right to have a letter forwarded, unopened, to the Minister for Health, the President of the High Court, the Registrar of Wards of Court, the health board, or the Inspector of Mental Hospitals. The minister may arrange for an examination of a patient by the Inspector of Mental Hospitals and may direct his discharge where justified. The President of the High Court may require the inspector to visit and examine any patient detained as a person of unsound mind and report to him.

(b) Any person may apply to the minister for an order for the examination, by two medical practitioners, of a patient detained and the minister may, if he thinks fit, on consideration of their report, direct the discharge of the patient.

(c) The act specifically requires that a patient who has recovered must be discharged.

(d) Penalties are imposed by the act for detention otherwise than in accordance with the provisions of the act.

(e) Any relative or friend of a person detained may apply for the discharge of a patient and, if the medical officer of the institution certifies that the patient is dangerous or otherwise unfit for discharge, an appeal lies to the minister.

Voluntary patients

A patient may, without the recommendation of a medical practitioner, apply to be admitted for treatment in a mental hospital as a voluntary patient. A person admitted in this way may leave the hospital at any time on giving three days' notice. Where a person is under sixteen years of age, application for admission must be made by his parent or guardian, and must be accompanied by a recommendation from a registered medical practitioner.

Special provisions on detention of psychiatric patients

Because of the nature of their illness, there are a number of special restrictions in connection with the keeping and treatment of psychiatric patients. To keep a person of unsound mind in an unregistered institution is an offence. Concealment of a patient in a mental hospital, assisting such a patient to escape and ill-treatment or neglect of a patient all carry heavy penalties and the use of mechanical means of restraining patients is subject to stringent regulation. The regulations require that 'patients in a mental institution shall be treated with all gentleness compatible with their condition, and restraint, when necessary, shall be as moderate, both in extent and duration, as is consistent with the safety and advantage of the patients'. Dietaries, bathing, visiting hours and correspondence are also among the subjects covered by the regulations.

The Inspector of Mental Hospitals

The Minister for Health is required to appoint a registered medical practitioner as Inspector of Mental Hospitals. The inspector has wide duties and powers in relation to the inspection of mental hospitals and the patients in them. He regularly visits each mental institution on a general inspection and may, at any time of the day or night, enter and inspect any such institution and examine any patient. All reasonable facililties for his inspections must be afforded to him. His annual reports, which he makes to the minister, are published.

Criminal lunatics

A criminal lunatic may be described as any person who, while in custody, has been certified to be insane in any of the following circumstances:

(a)   while on remand or awaiting trial;

(b)   while undergoing sentence either in a local or convict prison;

(c)   while awaiting the pleasure of the government, having been found insane by a jury on arraignment; or

(d)   while awaiting the pleasure of the government, having been found 'guilty but insane' by a jury.

252

Criminal lunatics are confined either in the Central Mental Hospital, Dundrum or in a district mental hospital, on the order of the Minister for Justice. A case defined as at (a) above must be sent to the district mental hospital serving the area where the person is in custody, while cases at (b) undergoing sentence in a convict prison must be sent to Dundrum when certified insane. The Minister for Justice has discretion to send other cases either to the district mental hospital or to Dundrum.

APPENDIX F

Registration of births, deaths and marriages: vital statistics

REGISTRATION

Two acts passed in 1863 – the Registration of Births and Deaths (Ireland) Act and the Registration of Marriages (Ireland) Act – saw the commencement of the present comprehensive system for the registration of births, deaths and marriages. Until then there was no civil registration of births or deaths in Ireland and the registration of marriages did not extend to marriages in Catholic churches (which were much more numerous than other forms of marriage). The system of registration established in 1863 has not been altered in any major respect up to the present. It is based on local registrars under the supervision of superintendent registrars, who, in turn, are under an tArd-Chlaraitheoir (the Registrar-General).

Registration of births
The local registrar has the duty of registering all births which take place in his district. He keeps the register in local premises and the informant attends there to give the information necessary for registration and to sign the register. The duty of doing this rests primarily on the parents and, in their default, on the occupier of the house where the child was born, on each person present at the birth and on the person in charge of the child. The information recorded is the date and place of the birth, the name and sex of the child, the name, surname and dwelling-place of the father, the

254

name, surname and maiden surname of the mother and the rank or profession of the father.

Each quarter, the registrar sends to the superintendent registrar (i.e. the health board) a copy of the entries made by him in his register. The superintendent checks and certifies these and sends them to Oifig an tArd-Chlaraitheora. The local registrar keeps the register-book until it is filled, when he sends it to the superintendent registrar for retention. The copies of the entries in the local registers which are received in Oifig an tArd-Chlaraitheora (the General Register Office) are indexed and micro-filmed.

Birth certificates

Birth certificates are issued by Oifig an tArd-Chlaraitheora, the superintendent registrars and the local registrars. The last-named can only issue certificates of comparatively recent registrations as their register books when completed are sent to the superintendent registrar. Any member of the public is entitled, on paying a fee, to a certified copy of an entry in a register.

Two forms of certificate are issued, the full certificate, which is a true copy of the entry and the short certificate, on which is shown only the name, surname, sex and date of birth of the person and the district of registration.

Certificates required for some special purposes such as to accompany applications for children's allowances and other social welfare benefits, are obtainable from local registrars and superintendent registrars at a special fee.

Registration of deaths and issue of death certificates

The duty of registering all deaths which take place in his district also falls on the local registrar. In the case of a death taking place in a house, the obligation to inform the registrar rests, in the order of priority shown, on:

(a) the nearest relatives of the deceased present at his death or in attendance during his last illness,

(b) every other relative living or being in the same district as the deceased,

(c) each person present at the death,

(d) the occupier of the house or hospital where the death took place,

(e) each other inmate of the house,

(f) the person causing the body to be buried.

255

Rather similar priorities of obligation to register apply where a death occurs or where a dead body is found elsewhere than in a house.

The items registered are the date and place of the death, the name, surname, sex, conjugal condition, age and occupation of the deceased and the cause of death. The cause of death is usually certified by the medical practitioner who attended the deceased in his last illness. Where a post mortem or an inquest has been held, a coroner's certificate as to the cause is sent to the registrar. The death registers are checked, copied and indexed in the same way as the registers of births.

Registration of marriages
Under the Marriages (Ireland) Act, 1844 the registration of marriages, other than those in Catholic churches, was initiated through specially-appointed local registrars of marriages. At the same time the office of the Registrar-General of Marriages was established. Copies of the local registers were sent to this office and central recording of these marriages commenced.

Registration through different channels of Catholic marriages was introduced in 1863, when it was arranged that a certificate signed by the priest, the parties to the marriage and the witnesses, would be sent to the registrar of births and deaths. He was required to keep a register of such marriages and subsequent steps as respects checking, copying, indexing and the issue of certificates were prescribed as for registers of births and deaths.

These parallel procedures for registration of marriages continue today. The form of the marriage register is, however, the same in each case, the particulars required being the date of the marriage and, for each of the contracting parties, the name and surname, date of birth, previous marital condition, occupation, place of residence before and after marriage, name and surname of father and name and maiden surname of mother.

VITAL STATISTICS

Statistics of births, deaths and marriages
The basic vital statistics are those of births, deaths and marriages. From the establishment of his office, the Registrar-General had the duty of publishing annual abstracts of these statistics. These Reports

of the Registrar-General are the sources of most of the vital statistics for the period up to 1952, when the Registrar-General was relieved of this duty. Under the Vital Statistics and Births, Deaths and Marriages Registration Act, 1952 (No. 8 of 1952), the Minister for Health was given power to compile and publish vital statistics and to do this, if he wished, through the agency of other government offices. This placed on a formal basis an arrangement under which the statistical work which stemmed from the registration system was done by the Central Statistics Office.

The Vital Statistics Regulations, 1954 (S.I. 280 of 1954)
From 1 January 1955, an improved system was introduced for collecting statistics of births and deaths. Before then only the information required to be given for registering a birth or death was available to the statistical service. This was not sufficient to allow for the production of some desirable statistical tables and indices. In relation to births, for example, it was not known what number of previous children there were in the family or what the mother's age was – both important factors in calculating fertility rates and making population forecasts.

Under the new system, statistical forms were introduced for completion by the informant at the registration of a birth or death. These forms provide for the items already required for registration and information to be used for the compilation of statistics. The complete list of relevant items on the birth form is:
(a)   date and place of birth of the child;
(b)   sex of the child;
(c)   name and dwelling place of the father;
(d)   occupation of the father;
(e)   date of birth of the mother;
(f)   dwelling place of the mother before the birth;
(g)   year of present marriage of the mother;
(h)   number of children of the mother by her present or any previous husband—
   (i)   born alive and still living,
   (ii)   born alive, but dead at the time the particulars are furnished.

The headings on the form for deaths are:
(a)   date and place of death;

(b)   name and home address of deceased person;
(c)   sex of deceased person;
(d)   whether the deceased person was married, widowed or single;
(e)   age of the deceased person (in hours if under one day, in completed days if under one month, in completed months if under one year and otherwise in completed years);
(f)   the occupation of the deceased person, or where the deceased person was a child, the occupation of the parent or guardian;
(g)   if the deceased person was a married or widowed female, the occupation of her husband.

The registrar verifies that the forms are properly completed and sends them to the Central Statistics Office.

Foetal deaths
The collection of information on foetal deaths is a feature of the vital statistics in most modern states. Comprehensive, systematic collection of these statistics commenced in Ireland from 1 January 1957 under the Vital Statistics (Foetal Deaths) Regulations, 1956 (S.I. No. 302 of 1956), of which the following sentences are a summary. When a foetal death occurs after the twenty-eighth week of pregnancy, the medical practitioner or midwife (or medical student or pupil midwife) is required to send information about it to the local medical officer. Forms for this purpose are provided by the health board. The headings under which information is given on the form are:
(a)   date and place of the confinement;
(b)   estimated period of gestation;
(c)   sex of the foetus;
(d)   putative cause of the foetal death;
(e)   name and normal dwelling place of mother;
(f)   date of birth of the mother;
(g)   year of present marriage of the mother;
(h)   number of previous children of the mother (by her present or any previous husband)—
    (i)   still living
    (ii) born alive but now dead;
(i)   number of previous foetal deaths (if any) as respects the mother.

The form is in two parts: that with the name and address of the mother is kept by the medical officer and he sends the remainder of the form to the Central Statistics Office. Statistics of foetal deaths are included in the Annual Reports on Vital Statistics (published by the Stationery Office).

APPENDIX G

Officers and servants of health boards

The provisions of the Health Act, 1970 (Chapter II of Part II), are summarised below and the minister's directions (as operative on 1 January, 1988) under these provisions are quoted, where appropriate.

CHIEF EXECUTIVE OFFICERS

The basic legal provisions on the office of chief executive officer of a health board are in section 13 of the 1970 act, primarily in subsection (1), which reads:

> There shall be appointed, in respect of each health board established under this Act, a person who shall be called and shall act as the chief executive officer of the board.

Section 13(2) relates to appointments of deputy chief executive officers (ordinarily selected by the chief executive officer himself from among the other officers of the board, but if the chief executive officer is temporarily unable to act, the chairman (or vice-chairman) of the board may appoint the deputy from among the other officers of the board). The minister may specify the classes of officers who may be appointed as deputy chief executive officer.

Subsection (4) states:

> A chief executive officer shall hold his office on such terms and conditions and shall perform such duties as the Minister from time to time determines.

When an office of chief executive officer is vacant, the minister may, after consultation with the chairman of the board (or in his absence, the vice-chairman) make a temporary appointment under section 13 (9). Selections for permanent appointments of chief

executive officers are made through the Local Appointments
Commission (section 15).

OTHER OFFICERS AND SERVANTS

Numbers and types
The general power for the appointment of other officers and
servants is in section 14(1) of the 1970 act which reads:
> In addition to the chief executive officer, there shall be
> appointed to a health board such and so many other officers
> and such and so many servants as the board from time to
> time determines in accordance with the directions of the
> Minister.

The general directions of the minister on this are:
> Where a health board makes a determination in respect of
> the number and type of appointments to be made it shall be
> on the basis that no appointments of officers will be made in
> respect of such determination until the Minister consents
> except:
> (a)   insofar as the determination relates to additional
>   appointments of a temporary nature which the chief
>   executive officer considers urgently necessary and which
>   are made for a period not exceeding four weeks and
> (b)   in such other cases as the minister may direct.

Appointments and terms and conditions
The appointment of officers and servants is a function of the chief
executive officer (section 14(2)). However, under subsection (5),
the chief executive officer must act in accordance with the directions
of the minister.

The directions of the minister on this are:
> The chief executive officer shall comply with the following
> provisions when making an appointment as an officer to
> which the Local Authorities (Officers and Employees) Acts,
> 1926, and 1940 do not apply.
> (a)   When the need to fill a vacancy arises an advertisement
>   shall be published as soon a possible in the public press
>   inviting applications from qualified persons and speci-
>   fying a closing date which allows a reasonable period
>   for potential candidates to inform themselves of the
>   particulars of the appointment and to apply in such

form as may be required. Completed application forms received after the date specified in the advertisement as the latest date for the receipt of completed application forms should not be considered and this should be clearly stated in the advertisements and on application forms. If it is intended to make more than one appointment, the advertisement should so indicate. If a panel is to be formed from which further appointments may be made if required during a period ahead, it should be so stated in the advertisement. All material circulated to candidates should contain a footnote indicating that canvassing will disqualify. Canvassing should be interpreted to comprehend all representations, written or oral.

(b) The selection of a candidate or candidates to be appointed or of the candidates to be placed in order of merit on a panel shall be by means of a selection procedure appropriate to the appointment having regard to the nature of the duties, the knowledge and experience necessary for the efficient performance of the duties and the qualifications for the appointment. Where the selection is not made on the results of a competitive examination, whether a general examination conducted by the Department of Education or an examination held specially on behalf of the health board, a suitably constituted interview board should be set up to assess the relative merits of candidates. A short list of candidates to attend before the interview board may be prepared by the latter from an examination of statements of qualifications furnished by candidates, at the request of the chief executive officer if he is satisfied that this course is justified, provided that the remaining candidates who possess the essential qualifications are notified accordingly.

(c) Subject to the paragraphs below appointments should be made by the chief executive officer in accordance with the results of the competitive examination or the recommendations of the interview board, except where it is necessary for him, on the ground of character, health, or previous employment record, to decide that a particular candidate is not suitable for employment.

The chief executive officer should satisfy himself on these points by having a medical examination carried out and by making appropriate enquiries. This sub-paragraph is without prejudice to existing directions in respect of disabled persons.

Where appointments in a particular grade are made frequently and a panel is formed for such appointments in accordance with the provision of paragraphs 2(a) and (b), either the number of names entered on the panel should be limited to the number of appointments which can be expected with reasonable certainty to be made within a year from the setting up of the panel or, if it is expedient to place a greater number of names on the panel to allow for wastage or for other reasons, the duration of the panel when it is being formed should be expressly limited to a specified period. Normally this period would be one year but it should not exceed two years.

Apart from the chief executive officer's responsibility to decide the suitability for appointment of every person appointed, the provisions need not be applied to:

(a) the appointment of trainee public health nurses following qualification and registration.

(b) the appointment of a person who is a member of a religious order in replacement of another member of that order who had been appointed without advertisement or competition.

Terms and conditions, remuneration, etc.

The remuneration and allowances of the chief executive officers are determined by the minister (section 13(5)). In practice, these determinations are now governed by recommendations made by the Review Body on Higher Remuneration in the Public Sector.

Terms and conditions, remuneration and allowances for other staff of health boards is governed by subsections (3) to (5) of section 14. The general directions issued by the minister under subsection (5) are:

The chief executive officer may assign remuneration according to their grades to officers and servants at the rates and on the conditions approved by the minister for the respective grades. The chief executive officer may also grant allowances to officers and servants at the rates and on the conditions approved by the Minister, not for named officers, but for general application or for application to members in general or of a particular grade e.g. allowances payable for acting as a substitute for an officer in a higher grade, allowances payable for possession of special qualifications or for special duties, including "on call" or "stand by" allowances.

Any variation in the rates of remuneration or allowances referred to at sub-paragraph (a) payable to an officer or servant or to officers or servants of a specified class, description or grade, and any new grant of an allowance to a named officer or any renewal of a grant to a named officer for a further period shall be subject to the approval of the Minister.

These directions are supplemented by detailed subsidiary directions on tenure of office, probation, sick pay and sick leave, annual leave, maternity leave, special leave, starting pay on promotion and travelling and subsistence allowances.

Job sharing and career breaks
Under a direction of the minister, health boards may introduce job sharing schemes for permanent staff except in respect of posts which are not suitable for job sharing. In general job sharing staff shall be entitled to similar conditions to persons employed on a full time basis. Applications by health board staff for career breaks should, as a general rule be granted provided that the needs of the service can be met.

Appeals to minister
Under section 14(6), there is appeal to the minister against a determination by the chief executive officer under subsection (3) or (4). The procedure for this, as laid down by the minister is:

Any officer of the health board who is aggrieved by a decision of his chief executive officer in relation to his terms and conditions of employment, duties, remuneration or allowances, may apply to the Minister to issue a direction to the chief executive officer in relation to such decision and the Minister may issue such direction as he considers appropriate to the chief executive officer in relation to such decision.

An officer who wishes to apply to the minister to issue a direction to the chief executive officer under section 14(6) of the Health Act, 1970 shall proceed as follows—

(i)   He shall prepare a statement in writing setting out the decision of the chief executive officer by which he is aggrieved and the ground on which he is so aggrieved;

(ii) He shall send the said statement by registered post to the minister together with a signed declaration that the facts contained in the said statement are true;

(iii) Before sending the said statement to the minister, he shall give or send by post written notice of the application to the chief executive officer together with a copy of the said statement.

Deputising arrangements
An officer under a health board may arrange for his duties to be performed for a specified period by a deputy nominated by him. The minister's consent is needed, or the consent of the chief executive officer given in accordance with any directions of the minister (section 14(7) and (8)).

Posts filled through Local Appointments Commission
Under section 15 of the 1970 act, the minister may specify offices (additional that of chief executive officer) to be filled by selection through the Local Appointments Commission, rather than by the selection process described above.

The minister's determination on this is as follows:

The Minister has determined, with the consent of the Local Appointments Commissioners, under section 15(1) of the Health Act, 1970 that the Local Authorities (Officers and Employees) Acts, 1926 and 1940 apply, without any modifications to —

(a) permanent appointments under a health board corresponding to appointments to the offices under a local authority referred to at Section 2(1)(b) of the Local Authorities (Officers and Employees) Act, 1926, as amended. Notwithstanding this, the Acts will not apply to any grade of social worker or such other paramedical grades which the Minister may determine, with the consent of the local Appointments Commission, from time to time,

(b) permanent appointments of health inspectors and promotional grades of health inspector,

(c) permanent appointments of chief nursing officers, assistant chief nursing officers, matrons, deputy matrons, assistant matrons, in all hospitals and institutions other than

(i) county homes and institutions providing accommodation for similar classes of persons, district hospitals and fever hospitals of less than 100 beds and

(ii) hospitals, other than those mentioned at sub-paragraph (i), in which a religious order is associated with the administration of the hospital.

(d) permanent appointments of matrons and assistant matrons in hospitals referred to at sub-paragraph (c)(ii), if (i) the appointment is in replacement of an officer who was appointed on the recommendation of the Local Appointments Commissioners or (ii), in any other case, if the appointment is not the appointment of a member of the religious order associated with the administration of the hospital in replacement of another member of that order who had been appointed without advertisement or competition,

(e) permanent appointments of superintendent public health nurses and senior public health nurses,

(f) permanent appointments of director of nursing and assistant director of nursing in centres for the mentally handicapped.

Delegation by chief executive officer
Section 16 allows the chief executive officer to delegate functions to other officers, subject to any directions in that respect which may be given by the minister. No such directions have been given.

Performance of duties by officers
Section 17 defines the relative roles of the health board, the chief executive officer and the other officers of the board. This section reads:

17. (1) In the performance of their duties, the chief executive officer and the other officers of a health board shall act in accordance with such decisions and directions (whether of a general or a particular nature, as, subject to subsection (3), are conveyed to or through the chief executive officer by the board, and in accordance with any such decisions and directions so conveyed of a committee to which functions have been delegated by the board.

(2) When the chief executive officer or another officer of a health board performs a duty in accordance with subsection (1), he shall be deemed to act on behalf of the board.

(3) The board shall not take any decision or give any direction in relation to any matter which under this Act or any other enactment is a function of the chief executive officer or of another officer of the board.

(4) The following functions relating to a health board shall be functions of the chief executive officer of the board:

    (a) any function specified by this Act or by any other enactment to be a function of the chief executive officer of the board,

    (b) any function with respect to a decision as to whether or not any particular person shall be eligible to avail himself of a service (including a service for the payment of grants or allowances), or as to the extent to which, and the manner in which, a person shall avail himself of any such service,

    (c) any function with respect to a decision as to the making or recovery of a charge, or the amount of any charge for a service for a particular person,

    (d) any function with respect to the control, supervision, service, remuneration, privileges or superannuation of officers and servants of the board,

    (e) such other functions as may be prescribed.

(5) Any dispute —

    (a) as to whether or not a particular function is a function of the chief executive officer, or

    (b) as to whether or not a particular function is a function of an officer of a health board other than the chief executive officer, shall be determined by the Minister.

Qualifications

Section 18 provides:

    The qualifications for appointment as an officer, or for continuing as an officer, under a health board shall be approved or directed by the Minister and, in the case of an office to be filled by selection by the Local Appointments Commissioners, after consultation with the Commissioners

In the case of consultant medical staffs and certain other staff in health board hospitals, Comhairle na nOspideal has a role in specifying qualifications, 'subject to any general requirements determined by the Minister' (section 41(1)(b)(ii) of the 1970 act)

The following are the directions by the minister under section 18 of the act:

1. Qualifications generally:
   (a) Except for the appointment of a registered medical practitioner in an additional temporary appointment in certain circumstances no person shall be appointed as an officer who does not possess the qualifications approved of or directed by the Minister for the appointment, subject to sub-paragraph (b).
   (b) Where the chief executive officer experiences difficulty in obtaining suitable persons possessing all the qualifications approved or directed by the Minister for appointments in a particular grade, he may make appointments on a temporary basis without reference to such qualifications insofar as they relate to age.

2. Qualifications for appointment as an officer:
   (a) The qualifications for appointment as an officer in an existing grade in which officers were transferred from the service of local authorities shall be the qualifications which applied to offices in that grade under local authorities immediately prior to the transfer. Where such qualifications contain an upper age limit and concede an exemption to existing pensionable officers such concession may be applied to existing pensionable officers of both health boards and local authorities in the State.
   (b) Where an appointment as an officer has to be made and no qualifications are applicable to such appointment in accordance with sub-paragraph (a) above, the qualifications proposed by the chief executive officer for the appointment shall be referred to the Minister for approval, together with particulars of the nature and extent of the duties for which the appointment is required and other relevant information in regard to

the appointment, and the qualifications for the appointment shall be as approved of or directed by the Minister.

(c) The provisions of sub-paragraphs (a) and (b) which relate to appointment of officers, need not be applied to future appointments in grades in which officers have been transferred from the service of local authorities and which had been re-classified under local authorities as grades in which further appointments of officers need not be made. The officers transferred in these grades were appointed prior to the re-classification and should continue as officers. Their replacements and any additional appointments in the grades concerned should not be made as appointments of officers.

3. Qualifications for continuing as an officer:

(a) Where the qualifications for appointment as an officer referred to in sub-paragraphs 2(a) and (b) include in any case a requirement that the person to be appointed be registered or entitled to be registered in (i) the General Register of Medical Practitioners for Ireland, (ii) the Register of Dentists for Ireland, or (iii) the Register of Nurses maintained by An Bord Altranais, the officer appointed in each case must be so registered while continuing as an officer.

(b) Every person appointed to an office in the psychiatric service of a health board as a general trained nurse must be registered in the Psychiatric Nurses Division of the Register of Nurses kept by An Bord Altranais before the expiration of a period of three years after his appointment as a condition of his continuing as an officer after the termination of such period.

Age limits for officers
Under section 19, there is an age limit of 65 years but the minister may by order fix a higher limit in any case. He has made such an order (the Health Officers (Age Limit) Order 1971 (S.I. No. 109 of 1971). It allows for an age higher than 65 years for each

(a) permanent officer who was transferred to the service of a health board on 1 April, 1971 and who immediately before such transfer was the holder of an amalgamated office where such office resulted from the amalgamation of an office of district medical officer of a dispensary district and another office,

(b) permanent officer who if he continues to hold office until he reaches a particular age higher than 65 will then and only then by law be entitled to or be capable of being granted a superannuation allowance on his resigning or otherwise ceasing to hold office, and

(c) permanent officer who is not by law entitled to or capable of being granted a superannuation allowance on his resigning or otherwise ceasing to hold office.

Superannuation
The Local Government (Superannuation) Act, 1956 (No. 10 of 1956) applies in relation to a health board and its officers and servants as if it were a local authority and they were officers and servants of a local authority (section 20 of the 1970 act).

Suspensions and removals
Sections 21 to 24 relate to the suspension or removal from office of a chief executive officer or another officer of a health board.

A chief executive officer may be suspended by the minister or by the board (by a resolution for the passing of which at least two-thirds of the members voted and of which at least seven days' notice was given to members). Suspensions may be terminated by the minister. The minister may remove a chief executive officer from office following a local inquiry (section 21).

For other officers, there are detailed provisions on suspensions by the chief executive officer (section 22) and removals from office (section 23 and 24). Further provisions are included in the Health (Removal of Officers and Servants) Regulation, 1971 (S.I. No. 110 of 1971) as amended by regulations of 1972 (S.I. No. 165 of 1972) and 1973 (S.I. No. 180 of 1973).

ARRANGEMENTS BETWEEN HEALTH BOARDS AND LOCAL AUTHORITIES

Section 25 of the 1970 act allows a health board to perform functions of a local authority on behalf of that authority (with the consent of the Minister for the Environment). It also allows duties relating to local authority functions to be assigned by the chief executive officer to an officer of the health board and vice versa in the case of health board functions and local authority officers.

CONTRACT ARRANGEMENTS

A health board may 'in accordance with such conditions (which may include provision for superannuation) as may be specified by the Minister, make and carry out an arrangement with a person or body to provide services under the Health Acts for persons eligible for such services (section 26(1))'. This is the legal basis for the arrangements with doctors and pharmacists under the general medical service.

ARRANGEMENTS BETWEEN HEALTH BOARDS

Two health boards 'may make and carry out an arrangement for the provision by one of them on behalf of and at the cost of the other of services under the Health Acts' (section 26(2)).

APPENDIX H

Part 1

ESTIMATED NON-CAPITAL EXPENDITURE BY PROGRAMMES AND SERVICES, 1985

Programme and service	Expenditure
	£m
1. Community protection programme	
1.1 Prevention of infectious diseases	5.163
1.2 Child health examinations	6.287
1.3 Food hygiene and standards	3.196
1.4 Drugs advisory service	0.520
1.5 Health education	2.229
1.6 Other preventive services	2.409
Programme total	19.804
2. Community health services programme	
2.1 General practitioner service (including prescribed drugs)	108.352
2.2 Subsidy for drugs purchased by persons ineligible under 2.1	6.600
2.3 Refund of cost of drugs for long-term illnesses (including hardship cases)	8.200
2.4 Home nursing services	20.060
2.5 Domiciliary maternity services	1.847
2.6 Family planning	0.125
2.7 Dental services	12.505
2.8 Ophthalmic services	3.826
2.9 Aural Services	0.807
Programme total	162.322

		£m
3.	Community welfare programme	
3.1	Cash payments and grants for disabled persons....	53.049
3.2	Mobility allowances for handicapped persons.......	0.341
3.3	Cash payments to persons with certain infectious diseases...	0.470
3.4	Maternity cash grants..	0.080
3.5	Domiciliary care allowances for handicapped children 5.060	
3.6	Cash payments to blind persons...........................	0.955
3.7	Home help services..	6.125
3.8	Meals-on-wheels services......................................	1.520
3.9	Grants to voluntary welfare agencies	9.400
3.10	Supply of milk to expectant and nursing mothers and children under five covered by medical cards	0.902
3.11	Pre-school support services..................................	0.514
3.12	Boarding-out of children......................................	2.529
3.13	Payments for children in residential homes	6.290
3.14	Welfare homes for the aged	7.449
3.15	Adoption services	0.530
	Programme total..	95.214

4.	Psychiatric programme:	
4.1	Service for diagnosis, care and prevention of psychiatric ailments...	146.666
	Programme Total..	146.666

5.	Programme for the handicapped	
5.1	Care in special homes for mentally handicapped....	69.975
5.2	Care of mentally handicaped persons in psychiatric hospitals	27.880
5.3	Care in day centres for mentally handicapped	6.898
5.4	Assessment and care of the blind............................	1,800
5.5	Assessment and care of the deaf.............................	0.550
5.6	Assessment and care of persons otherwise handicapped..	12.747
5.7	Rehabilitation service	2.995
	Programme total..	122.845

6. General hospital programme   £m
6.1 Services in regional hospitals 147.401
6.2 Services in public voluntary hospitals......................   252.060
6.3 Services in health board county hospitals
    and homes...   122.441
6.4 Contributions to patients in private hospitals..........   14.000
6.5 Services in district hospitals....................................   25.279
6.6 Services in health board long-stay hospitals............   59.013
6.7 Ambulance services...   17.018
    Programme total 637.212

7. General support programme:
7.1 Central administration..   7.138
7.2 Local administration (health boards) 33.304
7.3 Research 2.300
7.4 Superannuation..   13.125
7.5 Finance charges (including interest on borrowings,
    insurance), etc...   5.070
Programme total 60.937

Gross total for all programmes 1,245.000
Income (non-capital)
8.1 Charges for maintenance in private and semi-private
accommodation in public hospitals...............................   34.100
8.2 Other income*..   41.600
Total income..   75.700
Net total-all programmes 1,169.300

*Other income includes deductions from pay for emoluments and
superannuation, retentions from pensions, canteen receipts, payments
for agency services (health inspectors' services etc.) and investment
income (voluntary hospital and homes).

Source: Health Statistics 1986, Table J1.

Part 2

TRENDS IN NON-CAPITAL HEALTH EXPENDITURE 1971–1985

Year	Total expenditure Current Prices £mn	1971 Prices £mn	Expenditure per head of population Current Prices £mn	1971 Prices £mn	Percentage of GNP
1971–2	86.6	86.6	29.1	29.1	4.4
1972–3	108.1	99.4	35.8	32.9	4.6
1973–4	142.8	118.0	46.5	38.4	5.2
1974*	179.6	126.9	57.5	40.6	6.0
1975	242.6	141.7	76.4	44.6	6.5
1976	274.6	135.9	85.1	42.1	6.0
1977	328.0	142.8	100.2	43.6	5.9
1978	400.0	161.9	120.7	48.9	6.1
1979	505.0	180.5	149.9	53.6	6.6
1980	701.0	211.9	206.1	62.3	7.8
1981	822.7	206.6	238.9	60.0	7.6
1982	948.0	203.2	272.4	58.4	7.7
1983	1033.0	200.4	294.8	47.2	7.7
1984	1090.0	194.7	308.9	55.2	7.4
1985	1169.3	198.1	330.3	56.0	7.5

*Expenditure for the nine months to the end of 1974, converted to the annual equivalent.
Sources: Health Statistics, 1980 and 1986, Tables A4 and J13; *Administration Yearbook and Diary 1988*, Institute of Public Administration, page 384.

Bibliography

Stationery Office Publications

White Paper: Outline of Proposals for the improvement of the health services, 1947 (P 8400)

White Paper: Reconstruction and improvement of county homes, 1951 (Pr 756)

White Paper: Proposals for improved and extended health services, 1952 (Pr 1333)

Report of the Advisory Body on a Voluntary Health Insurance Scheme, 1956 (Pr 3571)

Report on the incidence of dental caries in school children, 1965 (Pr 8125)

Report of the Commission of Enquiry on Mental Handicap, 1965 (Pr 8234)

White Paper: The health services and their further development, 1966 (Pr 8653)

Report of the Commission of Enquiry on Mental Illness, 1966 (Pr 9181)

White Paper: The health services and their further development, 1966 (Pr 8653)

The Child Health Services – report of a study group, 1967 (Prl 171)

The Care of the Aged – report of an interdepartmental committee, 1968 (Prl 777)

Report of the Public Services Organisation Review Group, 1966–1969 (Prl 792)

Drug Abuse – report of a working party, 1971 (Prl 1774)

Psychiatric Nursing Services of Health Boards – report of a working party, 1973 (Prl 3445)

Restructuring the Department of Health – the separation of policy and execution, 1974 (Prl 3445)

The General Practitioner in Ireland – report of the

Consultative Council on General Practice, 1974 (Prl 3621)

Training and Employing the Handicapped – report of a working party, 1975 (Prl 4302)

Survey of the Workload of Public Health Nurses – report of a working group, 1975 (Prl 4315)

Report of the Committee on Non-accidental Injury to Children, 1976 (Prl 5538)

Some Major Issues in Health Policy – report no 29 of the National Economic and Social Council (NESC), 1977 (Prl 5821)

Universality and Selectivity: Strategies in Social Policy – report no 36 of NESC, 1978 (Prl 6416)

Report of the Working Party on General Nursing, 1980 (Prl 9156)

Report of the Review Body on Adoption Services, 1984 (Pl 2467)

Children's Dental Health in Ireland – a survey conducted by University College, Cork, 1984 (Pl 4530)

Health Services, 1983–1986

Community Care Services: an Overview – report no 84 of National Economic and Social Council, 1987 (Pl 4972)

Annual publications:

Health Statistics
Reports on Vital Statistics

Other publications

Adoption Board – annual reports

Barrington, Ruth: *Health, Medicine and Politics in Ireland, 1900–1970*, Institute of Public Administration, 1987

Browne, Noël: *Against the Tide,* Gill and Macmillan Ltd, 1986

Collis, WRF: *The State of Medicine in Ireland,* Parkside Press, 1943

Comhairle na nOspideal – periodic reports

Curry, John: *The Irish Social Services,* Institute of Public Administration, 1980

Dignan, Dr John, Bishop of Clonfert: *Social Security: outlines of a scheme of national health insurance,* 1944

General Medical Services (Payments) Board – annual reports

Health Research Board – annual reports (including reports of the former Medical Research Council and the Medico-Social Research Board)

National Drugs Advisory Board – annual reports

OECD, Paris: *Measuring Health Care,* 1960–1983
Financing and Delivery of Health Care, 1987

Robins, Joseph: *The Lost Children* (a study of charity children in Ireland, 1700–1900), Institute of Public Administration, 1980
Fools and Mad (a history of the insane in Ireland), Institute of Public Administration, 1986

Roche, Desmond: *Local Government in Ireland.* Institute of Public Administration, 1982

Tussing, Dale: *Irish Medical Care Resources: An Economic Analysis,* Economic and Social Research Institute, 1985

Voluntary Health Insurance Board – annual reports

Whyte, John: *Church and State in Modern Ireland, 1923–1970,* Gill and Macmillan, Ltd, 1971

Index

279

Costello, John A, 33
cottage hospitals, 121
Council of Europe, 151–2
County and City Infirmary,
    Waterford, 120
county boards of assistance, 25
county borough corporations, 19
county councils, 11, 19, 41, 42
    school medical services, 25
county homes, 21, 22, 36, 104, 112
county hospitals, 28, 116, 117–18,
    125
    in 1975 plan, 49, 125–6
    administration of, 21, 41–2
    recommendations, 124, 125
county infirmaries, 2
County Management Act, 1940, 26
county management system, 26–7
county medical officers of health,
    26, 28
Croom Orthopaedic Hospital, Co
    Limerick, 118

Dail Eireann
    and health services, 19–20, 25,
        135
    Select Committee on the Health
        Services, 34, 48
D'Alton, Cardinal, 33
Dangerous Drugs Act, 1934, 74
day care centres, 102
de Valera, Eamonn, 33
deaf, care of, 114
Dental Board, 28, 159
Dental Council, 159
dental services, 53–4, 69, 92–4, 146
dentistry, 15
dentists, 157, 159–60
Dentists Act, 1985, 50
Desmond, Barry, 50, 54, 109
Desmond, Eileen, 50
dieticians, 165
Dignan, Dr John (Bp Clonfert),
    31, 37

diphtheria immunisation, 24, 41,
    71
disabled, care of, 69, 114–15
    allowances, 97, 98
    supply of appliances, 87
disadvantaged children, 69, 100–2
dispensary service, 26, 31, 45, 48,
    51–2
    19th c, 3–5, 14, 15
    1900–45, 23
    1945–65, 36–7
    eligibility, 64
dispensing opticians, 164–5
district hospitals, 21, 41–2, 116,
    118, 125, 198
Dr Steevens' Hospital, Dublin, 119,
    123, 126
doctors
    see general practitioners; hospital
        consultants
drug abuse, 47, 49, 54, 69, 74–6,
    108, 199
drug addiction, 108
drugs, medical, 73
    Appendix C, 227–31
    control of, 52, 69, 75, 153, 156–7
    dispensing of, 85–6, 163
    improvements in, 70
    long-term illness, 87–8
    and mental illness, 36
    quality of, 74
    refund scheme, 87
    tuberculosis, 32
Dublin, Co
    county management system, 26
    eligibility, 37
    health authority, 42–3
Dublin, Co Dublin
    eligibility, 37
    health officers, 8
    hospitals, 2, 121, 122
    hospitals plan, 126
    regional hospital board, 59
Dublin Dental Hospital Board, 160
Dublin Health Authority, 59

Dublin House of Industry, 120
Dun Laoghaire Borough Council,
43
Dun Laoghaire Corporation, 141

Eastern Health Board, 52, 55, 108,
141
and drug abuse, 76
Education, Department of, 100
education, in workhouses, 12
electoral franchise, 13
eligibility, 63–7, 203
Appendix A, 207–8
categories of, 65–7
contributions, 61
for dispensary service, 31, 36–7
extension of, 33, 35, 45, 49
full, 63–4
limited, 65
means test, 38
emigration, 14, 152–3
Employment Equality Act, 1977,
170
Environment, Department of the,
70
epilepsy, 108
estate duty grant, 11
European Communities Act, 1972,
164
European Communities
(Proprietary Medicinal
Products) Regulations, 1974,
75
European Community, 75, 132
doctors in, 159
health finance, 175
hospital comparisons, 128–9
pharmacists in, 163–4
Social Fund, 115
Eurostat, 183
Exchequer, role of, 201–2
Eye, Ear and Throat Hospital,
Cork, 126

family planning services, 50, 69,
90–1
Famine, Great, 7, 14
Federation of Irish Chemical
Industries, 85
fever hospitals, 2, 116, 118
Fianna Fail, 30, 33, 34, 48
finance, 21, 105, 175–85, 195
19th c, 11–12
1900–45, 27
1945–65, 43, 44
1965–87, 47, 48, 57, 60–1
Appendix H, 272–5
capital, 183
cash benefits, 97–9
child care service, 101–2
future of, 200–5
general medical service, 86–7
health contributions, 184
hospital care service, 116
international comparisons, 181–
83, 196–7
non-capital expenditure, 175–83
percentage of GNP, 179
rise in costs, 179–81
sources of, 175–6, 200–1
Finance, Department of, 48–9
Fine Gael, 34, 49
Finglas West industrial school, 100
Finland, 182, 199
Fitzgerald, Professor Patrick, 123
Fitzgerald Report, 52–3, 59, 119–
20, 123–25
Fitzpatrick, David, 20
fixed amount grant, 27
Flanagan, Sean, 48, 123
fluoridation, 53–4, 93–4
food additives, 153
Appendix C, 223–5
Food and Agriculture
Organisation, 153
food hygiene, 8, 30, 69, 73, 74
Appendix C, 216–22
inspectors, 165
and local authorities, 41

Misuse of Drugs Acts
1977, 49, 50, 54, 74, 76
1984, 74, 76
Appendix C, 231–3
mobility allowances, 97
Monkstown Hospital, Co Dublin, 121
mortality rates
1900–45, 28–9
infectious diseases, 70
19th c, 14
tuberculosis, 32, 72
mother and child scheme, 32–3, 45
municipal corporations, 11

National Children's Hospital, Harcourt St, 120, 123, 126
National Co-ordinating Committee on Drug Abuse, 75
National Council for Educational Awards, 173
National Drugs Advisory and Treatment Centre, Jervis St, 75–6
National Drugs Advisory Board, 55, 75, 139, 148
National Health Council, 40–1, 138–9
National Health Insurance Society, 24, 31
National Insurance Bill, 1911, 18–19
National Maternity Hospital, Holles St, 122
National Medical Rehabilitation Centre, Dun Laoghaire, 115
National Rehabilitation Board, 95, 115, 149, 166
National Rehabilitation Centre, 122
national schools
medical examinations, 19, 78
National Social Service Council, 53
National University of Ireland, 27, 158, 160

Navan Orthopaedic Hospital, Co Meath, 118
non-teaching hospitals, 121
North Infirmary, Cork, 120, 126
Notification of Births (Extension) Act, 1915, 19
nurses, 160–2
registration of, 22, 161–2
training of, 13, 28, 173
Nurses Act, 1985, 50, 160
Nursing Board, 160–1
nursing services, 88–9
home nursing, 69

occupational therapists, 166
Offences Against the Person Act, 1861, 91
O'Hanlon, Rory, 51
O'Higgins, Kevin, 21
O'Higgins, T F, 34, 44, 48, 186
O'Malley, Donogh, 48
ophthalmic opticians, 164–5
ophthalmic services, 69, 94
opticians, 164–5
Opticians Act, 1956, 164
Organisation for Economic Co-operation and Development, 182, 196
orphanages, 101
orthopaedic hospitals, 116, 118, 121–2
Our Lady of Lourdes Hospital, Drogheda, 121
Our Lady's Hospital, Crumlin, 122
out-patient services, 67
charges for, 128
psychiatric, 36, 107
recommendations, 124
and VHI, 190

panel scheme, 18–19
pensions *see* superannuation
personnel, 155–73
1900–45, 27–8
continuing training, 172–3